CLEAN EATING
28-DAY PLAN

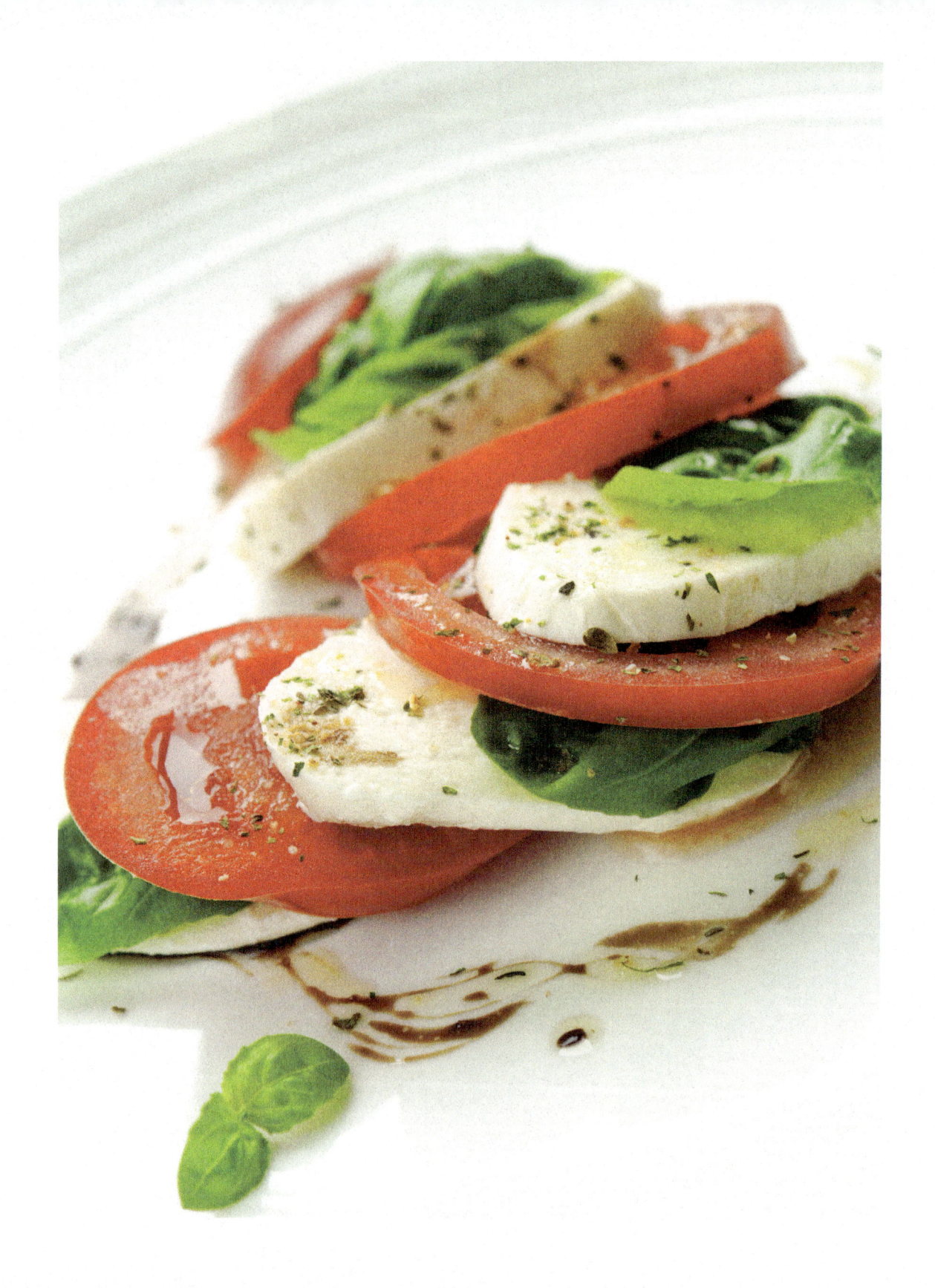

CLEAN EATING
28-DAY PLAN

A Healthy Cookbook and 4-Week Plan for Eating Clean

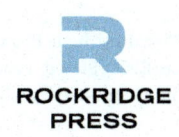

ROCKRIDGE PRESS

Copyright © 2014 by Rockridge Press, Berkeley, California

No part of this publication may be reproduced, stored in a retrieval system or transmitted in any form or by any means, electronic, mechanical, photocopying, recording, scanning or otherwise, except as permitted under Sections 107 or 108 of the 1976 United States Copyright Act, without the prior written permission of the Publisher. Requests to the Publisher for permission should be addressed to the Permissions Department, Rockridge Press, 918 Parker St., Suite A-12, Berkeley, CA 94710.

Limit of Liability/Disclaimer of Warranty: The Publisher and the author make no representations or warranties with respect to the accuracy or completeness of the contents of this work and specifically disclaim all warranties, including without limitation warranties of fitness for a particular purpose. No warranty may be created or extended by sales or promotional materials. The advice and strategies contained herein may not be suitable for every situation. This work is sold with the understanding that the publisher is not engaged in rendering medical, legal or other professional advice or services. If professional assistance is required, the services of a competent professional person should be sought. Neither the Publisher nor the author shall be liable for damages arising herefrom. The fact that an individual, organization or website is referred to in this work as a citation and/or potential source of further information does not mean that the author or the Publisher endorses the information the individual, organization or website may provide or recommendations they/it may make. Further, readers should be aware that Internet websites listed in this work may have changed or disappeared between when this work was written and when it is read.

For general information on our other products and services or to obtain technical support, please contact our Customer Care Department within the U.S. at (866) 744-2665, or outside the U.S. at (510) 253-0500.

Rockridge Press publishes its books in a variety of electronic and print formats. Some content that appears in print may not be available in electronic books, and vice versa.

TRADEMARKS: Rockridge Press and the Rockridge Press logo are trademarks or registered trademarks of Callisto Media Inc. and/or its affiliates, in the United States and other countries, and may not be used without written permission. All other trademarks are the property of their respective owners. Rockridge Press is not associated with any product or vendor mentioned in this book.

ISBN: Print: 978-1-62315-423-3 | eBook: 978-1-62315-421-9

Photo credits: Magdalena Paluchowska/Stockfood, p. xii; Eising Studio–Food Photo & Video/Stockfood, p. 57; Sporrer/Skowronek/Stockfood, p. 86; Eising Studio–Food Photo & Video/Stockfood, p. 110; Oliver Brachat/Stockfood, p. 126; Tim Winter/Stockfood, p. 150; Studio Lipov/Stockfood, p. 164; all other photographs www.shutterstock.com.

Quick-Start Guide

Review
Foods to eat. See page 7.

Identify
Foods to avoid and purge from your kitchen. See page 11.

Stock
Clean foods in your pantry. Find a list of everything you need on page 22.

Shop
For your first week of clean eating. See page 37.

Cook
Recipes begin on page 59.

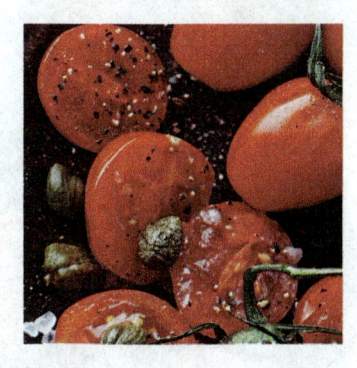

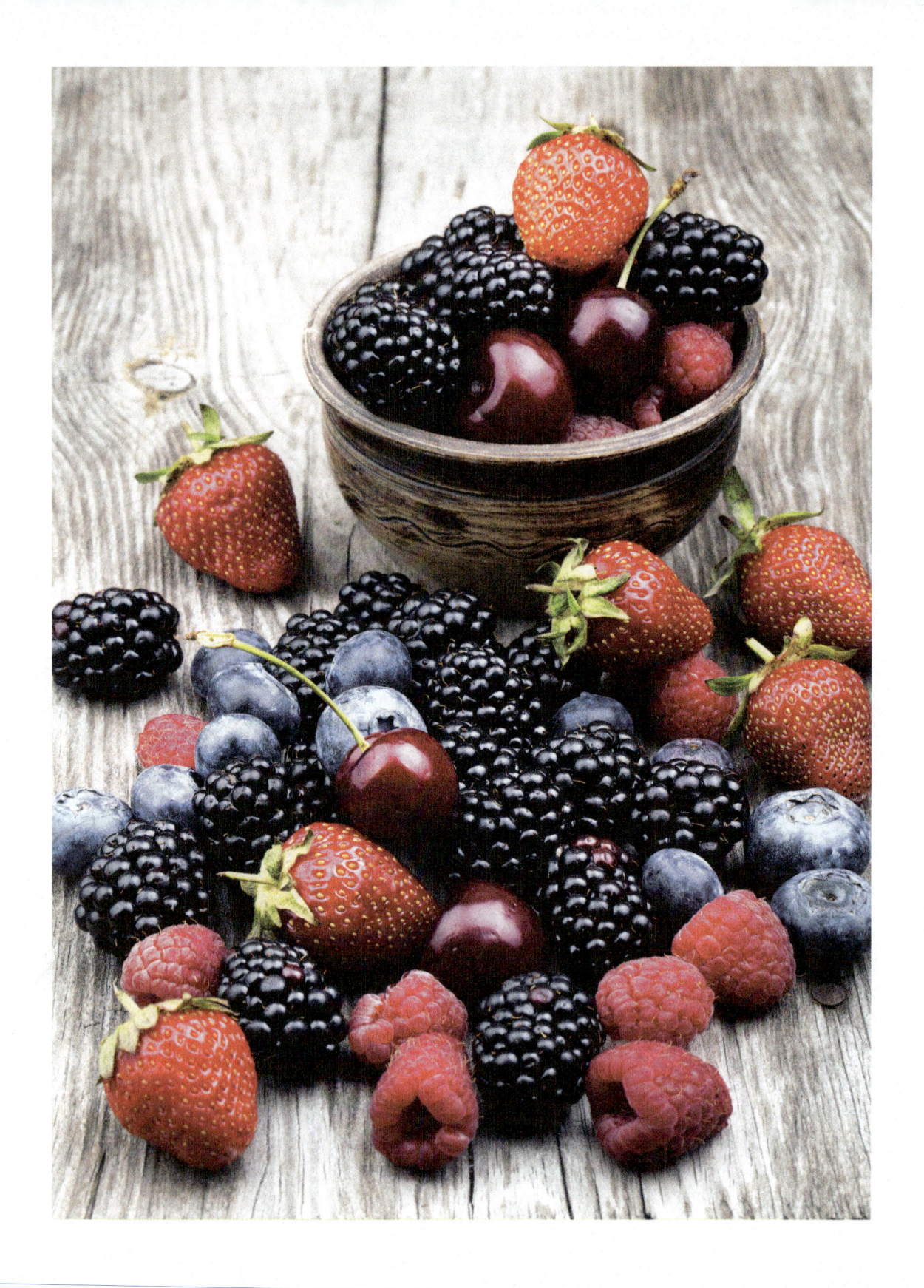

Contents

Introduction xiii

Part One: Getting Started

1. What Is Clean Eating? 1

2. How to Use the Meal Plan 17

3. Week-by-Week Clean Eating Meal Plans 31
Week One 33   Week Two 39   Week Three 45   Week Four 51

Part Two: Clean Eating Recipes

4. Breakfast

Ginger Berry Smoothie 60
Homemade Cinnamon Granola 61
No-Bake Coconut Granola Bars 63
Overnight Cinnamon Oatmeal 65
Protein-Packed Freezer Waffles (or Pancakes) 66
Whole-Wheat Maple Cinnamon Rolls 68
Whole-Wheat Blueberry Muffins with Cinnamon-Sugar Topping 70
Sweet Quinoa Breakfast Cups 72
Banana Blueberry Whole-Grain Pancakes 74
Red Pepper, Spinach, and Goat Cheese Frittata Bites 76
Scrambled Egg, Goat Cheese, and Cherry Tomato Pita Sandwich 77
Breakfast Tacos with Green Chiles, Goat Cheese, and Salsa Verde 79
Poached Eggs in Spicy Tomato Sauce 81

Poached Eggs and Asparagus on Whole-Grain Toast   82
Bacon-Crusted Mini Quiches with Mushrooms and Greens   84

5. Lunch

Fresh Herb Frittata with Peas, Bacon, and Feta Cheese   88
Caprese Salad with Balsamic Vinaigrette   90
Spicy Southwestern Corn and Bean Salad   91
Roasted Butternut Squash Salad with Goat Cheese, Walnuts,
 and Balsamic Vinaigrette   92
Mediterranean Chickpea Salad with Red Bell Peppers and Feta Cheese   94
Brussels Sprouts and Chickpea Salad with Dried Cranberries   95
Quinoa Salad with Cannellini Beans, Tomatoes, and Lemon Vinaigrette   96
Brown Rice and Black Bean Salad with Spinach and Lemon Vinaigrette   97
Shrimp Salad over Greens with Yogurt Dressing   98
Spinach Salad with Chicken and Sun-Dried Tomato and Basil Vinaigrette   99
Garden Salad with Chicken and Balsamic Vinaigrette   100
Roasted Vegetable Pitas with Pesto Mayonnaise   101
Egg Salad Sandwich with Greek Yogurt and Dill   102
Curried Chicken Salad Lettuce Wraps with Homemade Mayonnaise   103
Spiced Chicken Wraps with Yogurt Dressing and Fresh Mint   104
Korean Pork Lettuce Wraps with Fresh Herbs   105
Smoky Red Lentil Soup with Greens   106
Spicy Black Bean Soup with Vegetables   108

6. Snacks

Pineapple Coconut Trail Mix   112
Peanut Butter Energy Bites   113
Tropical Sweet Bars   114
Apple Walnut Bars   115
Banana Nut Bread   116
Honey Sesame Crackers   118
Creamy Peanut Butter–Yogurt Dip   119
Spiced Roasted Chickpeas   120
Smoky-Sweet Chili Almonds   121

Basil Garlic Zucchini Chips   122
Oven-Baked Sweet Potato Fries   123
Pesto White Bean Spread   124

7. Vegetarian Dinners

Stacked Eggplant Parmesan   128
Vegetarian Chili with Pinto Beans   130
Pumpkin and Chickpea Curry   132
Chickpea Tostadas with Cashew Cheese   133
Spinach and White Bean Enchiladas with Cashew Cheese   135
Roasted Butternut Squash and Black Bean Burritos with Goat Cheese   137
Balsamic-Roasted Vegetables with Quinoa   139
Quinoa-Stuffed Peppers with Black Beans and Yogurt Dressing   141
Whole-Wheat Pasta with Chickpeas and Spicy Tomato Sauce   143
Vegetable Stew   144
Risotto with Mushrooms and Peas   146
Brussels Sprouts Hash with Caramelized Onions and Poached Eggs   148

8. Fish and Seafood Dinners

Grilled Shrimp Tacos with Salsa Verde and Spicy Slaw   152
Garlic-Broiled Shrimp and Peppers over Quinoa   154
Seared Ahi Tuna with Chili-Lime Aioli   156
Balsamic-Glazed Wild Salmon with Garlicky Sautéed Spinach   157
Red Snapper with Spiced Pumpkin Seed Butter   159
Oven-Roasted Monkfish and Asparagus with Romesco Sauce   160
Soy-Glazed Cod with Japanese-Style Pickled Cucumber   161
Italian Fish Stew   163

9. Meat and Poultry Dinners

Roasted Chicken and Vegetables   166
Chicken Enchiladas Verdes with Goat Cheese   168
Tandoori-Spiced Chicken Breast with Crisp Cucumber Salad   170
Roasted Chicken Breasts with Mustard and Greens   172
Thai-Style Curried Chicken Burgers   174

Chicken and White Bean Chili   175
Turkey Meatballs with Whole-Wheat Spaghetti
   and Spicy Tomato Sauce   177
Lamb Loin Chops with Yogurt-Mint Sauce   179
Goat Cheese and Spinach–Stuffed Pork Chops   181
Grilled Pineapple and Pork Skewers   183
Korean Stir-Fried Pork with Brown Rice   184
Pork Fried Brown Rice with Pineapple and Cashews   186
Bacon-Wrapped Meatloaf   188
Sesame-Soy Marinated Flank Steak with Wasabi-Spiked
   Cauliflower Purée   190
Quinoa Fried "Rice" with Flank Steak and Peas   192

10. Dessert

Yogurt Blueberry Ice Pops   196
Banana Maple Nut "Ice Cream"   197
Cocoa Almond Pudding   198
Peanut Butter Oatmeal Cookies   199
Apple Crisp with Fresh Ginger   200
Berry Crumb Cake   202
Banana Chocolate Tart   204
Molten Chocolate Cakes   206
Rich Chocolate Fudge   207
Mini Cheesecakes in Caramel Sauce   208

11. Kitchen Staples—Condiments, Sauces, and Dressings

Guacamole   212
Pico de Gallo   213
Balsamic Vinaigrette   214
Lemon Vinaigrette   215
Yogurt Dressing   216
Homemade Mayonnaise   217
Salsa Verde   218

Fresh Basil Pesto   219
Romesco Sauce   220
Spicy Tomato Sauce   221
Chicken Broth   222
Vegetable Broth   223
Cashew Cheese   224
Homemade Almond Milk   225
Whipped Coconut Cream   226

Appendix A: 10 Tips for Eating Out   227
Appendix B: Conversion Tables   229
Resources   230
References   231
Recipe Index   233
Index   235

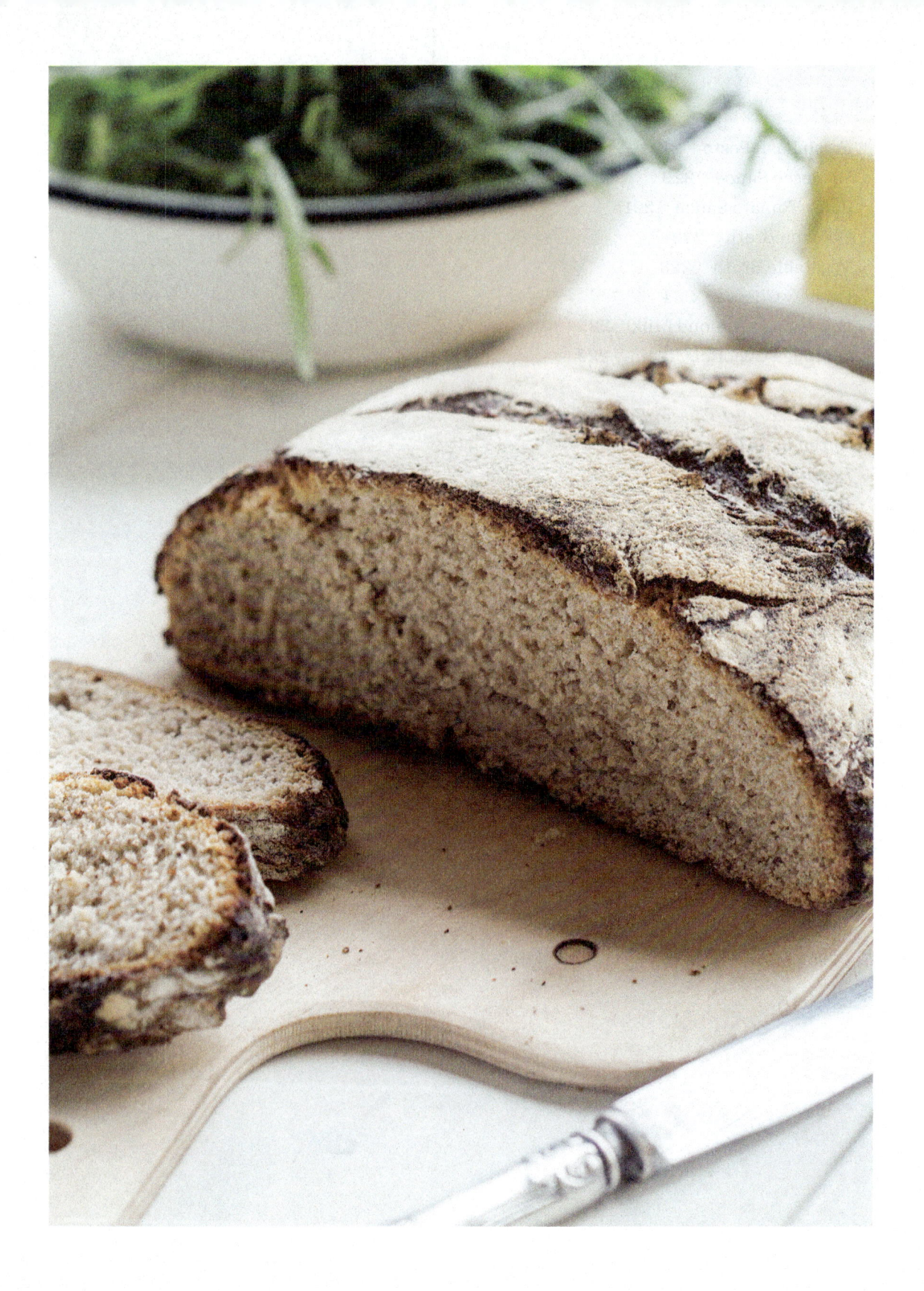

Introduction

Imagine that you're opening your refrigerator. What's in it? Maybe some fresh fruit, greens that look a bit wilted, cheeses of the "string" and "block" variety, a salmon steak or two, and some seasonal vegetables. Sure, it's all food, and good food, but what goes with what—and quickly? Do you see a healthful meal just waiting to be made, or do you start to think about ordering takeout?

Since you're reading this book, it's clear you have some health goals: a desire to eat better, or to lose weight, or maybe to ward off modern diseases (diabetes, heart disease, cancer, and other diseases with known dietary risk factors). "Clean eating" is a dietary concept that appeals to many because it is rooted in good old-fashioned common sense and sound nutritional science. Clean eating simply describes a healthful lifestyle that focuses on eating nutritious foods—specifically, foods that are whole, natural, unprocessed, unadulterated, and organic when available. And so it is about feeling good about the foods you eat.

But what about finding time in your daily life to make meals from whole foods that, well, must be *made*? The clean eating way is not about popping a Lean Cuisine in the microwave. It will put you in charge of your health and your meals, and that is incredibly empowering. But it also puts you in charge of preparing those meals. In truth, it can be tough to get started. That's where this book comes in. It was written specifically to help you make changes in your diet without having to worry about what to buy at the grocery store and what to cook. You are provided with a detailed four-week meal plan that takes the planning out of your meals. It tells you exactly what ingredients should be in your pantry, provides lists of what to buy at the market each week, and leaves you to cook and enjoy real, healthful, clean food.

In addition to helping you learn the basic principles of clean eating and how to incorporate them into your daily life, this book also provides:

- Advice on reading food labels, eating in restaurants, grocery shopping, stocking your pantry, useful kitchen gear, and cooking techniques
- A detailed four-week meal plan—three meals for each day, as well as snack suggestions—that will help you kick-start your new clean eating lifestyle, get on the right track, and stay the course for the long haul
- More than 100 recipes for delicious, nutritious, healthy, and clean dishes for every meal of the day

Don't worry if you aren't ready to completely change the way you eat every minute of every day. Eating clean doesn't have to be an all-or-nothing proposition from the get-go. You can start slowly by reducing the worst offenders your diet—such as those with artificial flavors and sweeteners, refined sugar and flour, and excess salt—and replacing them, one meal at a time, with fresh, whole foods like organic vegetables, fruits, meats, dairy products, and whole grains. But since you'll be eating foods you love and enjoying your meals, it will be easier than you might think to adapt the clean eating lifestyle for the long term. Soon you'll be aglow with the good health that results from a clean diet.

PART ONE
Getting Started

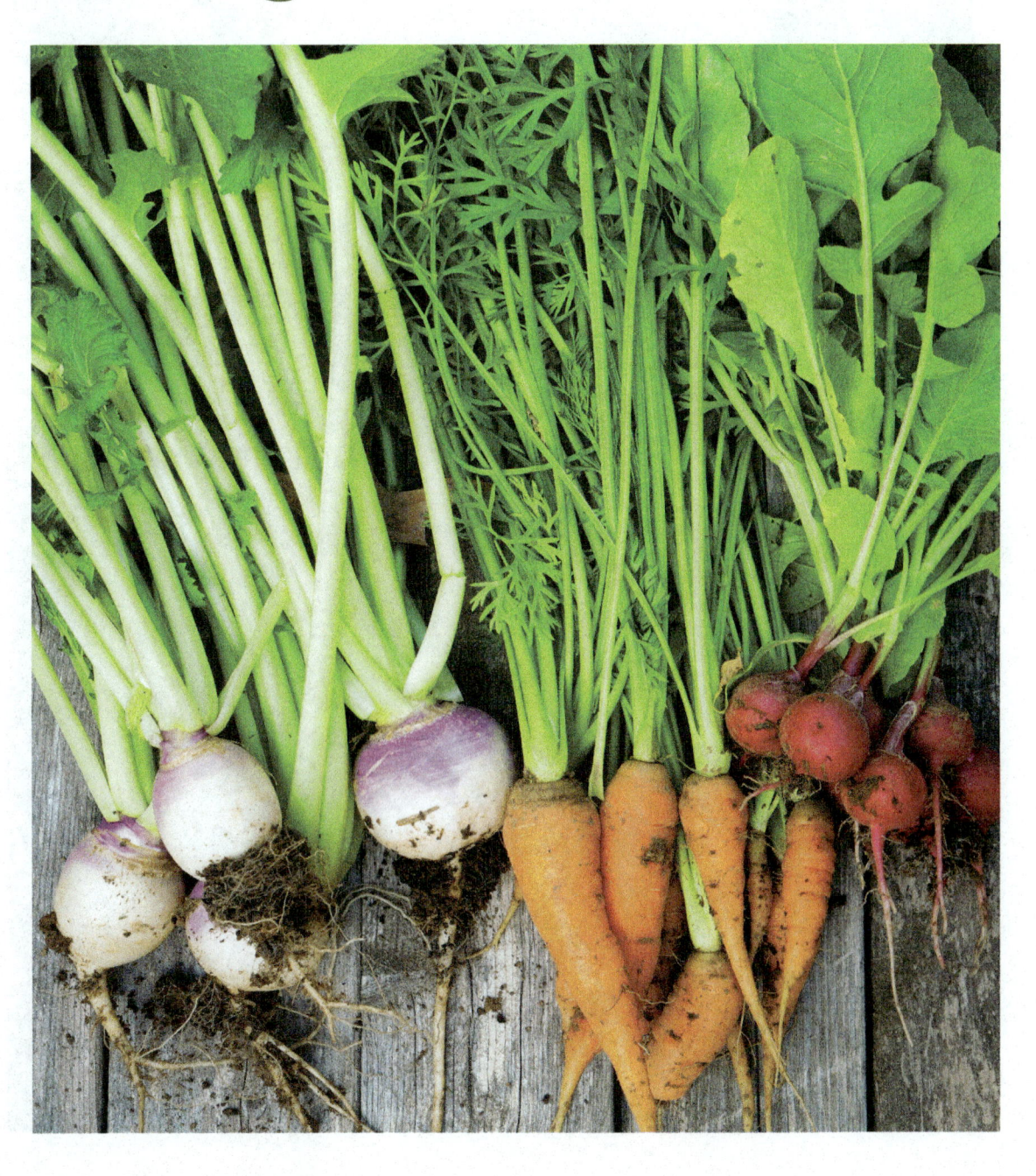

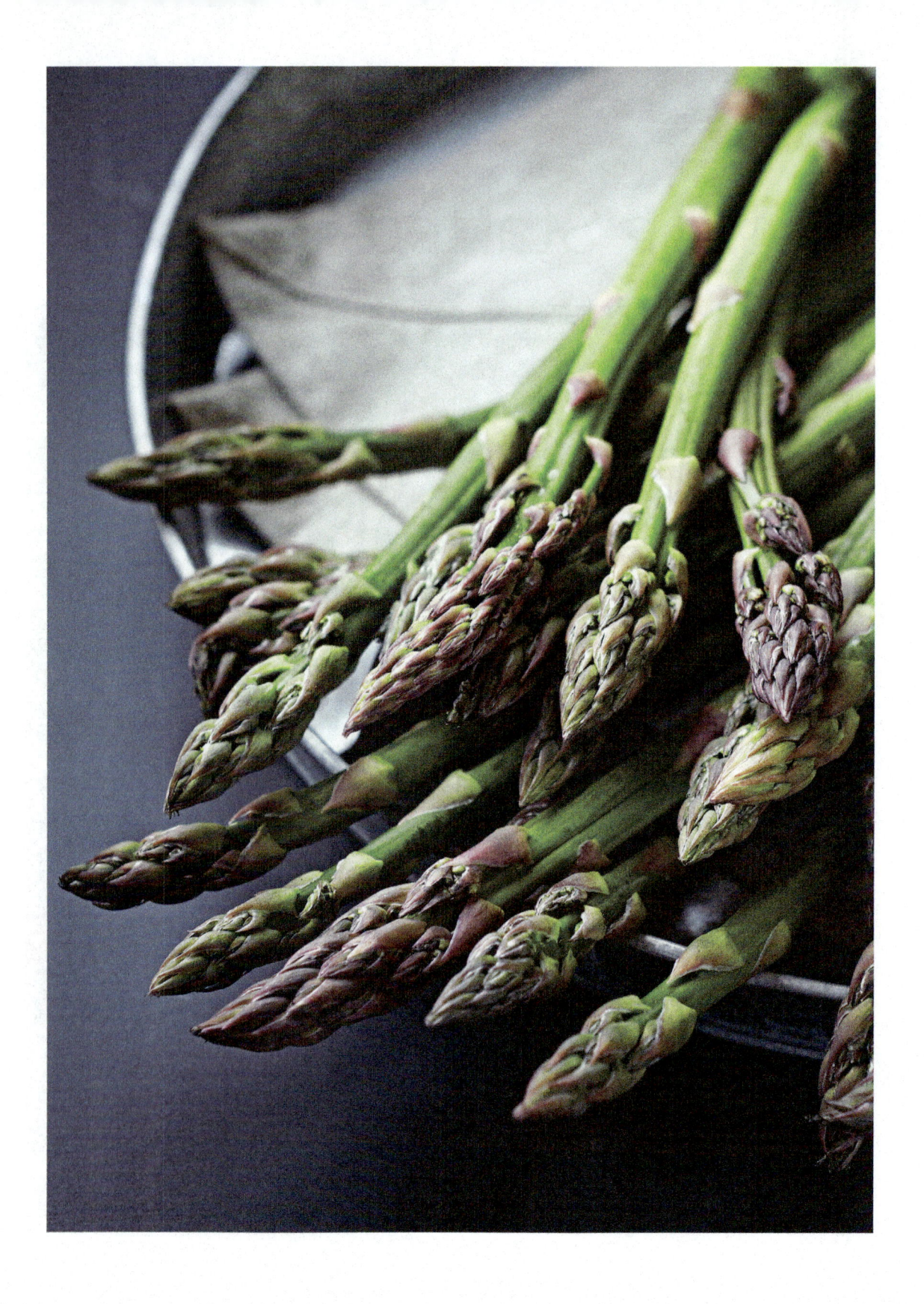

What Is Clean Eating?

Eating clean involves choosing foods that are as close to the way nature made them as possible. Think of a whole, fresh, crisp apple versus a bowl of canned applesauce or a glass of apple juice. Think of a bowl of steamed quinoa studded with fresh vegetables and herbs instead of packaged pasta with jarred tomato sauce. Think of a ripe banana and a handful of walnuts rather than a store-bought granola bar.

When you adopt the clean eating diet, you'll eliminate processed foods, such as refined sugar and flour and foods with artificial additives like colors, flavors, sweeteners, and preservatives. Instead, you'll eat the most healthful natural and organic foods available, including vegetables, fruits, whole grains, meats, and dairy products.

Much more than a diet, clean eating is a lifestyle that is accessible to anyone. And best of all, the principles are flexible and easily adapted to your individual circumstances.

Why Choose to Eat Clean?

Clean eating is not a short-term diet designed to help you shed a few pounds in the weeks leading up to your high school reunion. Many people do find that they lose weight effortlessly when they adopt clean eating, but the health advantages go way beyond that.

Heavily processed foods that are loaded with sugar, refined flours, and artificial colors and flavors are often nearly devoid of nutrition. By cutting the junk from your diet, you will boost the good food you're eating, including whole grains, which provide heart-healthy fiber, vitamins, and minerals; fresh fruits and veggies, which provide oodles of vitamins as well as fiber; protein-rich lean meats; and calcium-rich dairy products. It is fair to say that adopting this approach will leave you feeling healthier than before. Along with the specific benefits detailed here, clean eating will help you *feel better*.

By following a clean eating diet you will:

- **Boost your energy.** Fresh, nutrient-dense foods nourish your body and provide energy. To access fuel and function properly, your cells need certain nutrients—such as B-complex vitamins and iron—that come from the types of whole foods featured in the clean eating diet.

- **Strengthen your immunity.** Beta-glucans, a type of fiber that is found in the bran of many whole grains, especially oats and barley, possess antimicrobial and antioxidant qualities that boost immunity, expedite healing, and may improve the function of antibiotics. A study published in the medical journal *Surgery* found that beta-glucans significantly boosted the human immune system's response to bacterial infection. Eating whole, unprocessed grains increases your intake of these substances, making you more resistant to illness.

- **Regulate your blood sugar.** Fiber in whole grains, fruits, and vegetables helps regulate your blood sugar and eliminate blood sugar spikes and the fatigue that comes after them. According to the Mayo Clinic's guide to nutrition and healthy eating, dietary fiber can slow the absorption of sugar and help improve blood sugar levels. It can even help people with diabetes manage the symptoms of the disease. A fiber-rich diet may also lessen the risk of developing type 2 diabetes.

- **Lose weight.** Piling on the fresh veggies and fruits is a surefire way to fill up without overdoing it on calories. With produce, you get lots of vitamins and minerals that will nourish your body. You'll also boost your intake of dietary fiber, which makes you feel full faster and stay full longer—a key to weight loss. High-fiber foods also tend to be less calorie-dense and require more chewing. This extra time spent lingering over your meal gives your body a chance to feel satisfied, and so you're less likely to eat more calories than your body needs. According to WebMD and Eatright.org, if you start your day with a breakfast that includes fiber-rich whole grains, you'll be less likely to feel hungry before lunch.

> ### What Are Whole Grains and Why Are They Good for You?
>
> Grains are the seeds of cereal plants such as wheat, oats, barley, amaranth, quinoa, teff, rye, and others. Grains are harvested whole, including all parts of the seed: the bran (the outer skin of the seed, which contains antioxidants, B vitamins, and fiber), the germ (the heart of the seed, which contains B vitamins, protein, minerals, and healthful fats), and the endosperm (the bulk of the seed that provides the fuel that allows the germ to grow and develop, and is made up primarily of carbohydrates and proteins.)
>
> When whole grains are refined, they are stripped of the bran and the germ, leaving only the endosperm. As a result, they lose one-quarter of their protein and most of their fiber, vitamins, and minerals. The bottom line is that whole grains contain far more nutrients than refined grains. They can be cooked and eaten whole or they can be milled into flour and used to bake bread and other grain-based products.

- **Improve your cardiovascular health.** Fresh whole fruits and vegetables are loaded with vitamin C, which improves the function of your blood vessels. A diet rich in foods that contain vitamin C reduces your risk of coronary heart disease, stroke, high blood pressure, and immune deficiencies. In fact, according to a study by Mark Moyad, MD, at the University of Michigan, a higher blood level of vitamin C may be a reliable indicator for overall good health.
- **Lower your cholesterol.** According to the Harvard School of Public Health, a diet rich in unsaturated, or "good," fats—the type found in nuts, avocados, and olive oil—can improve blood cholesterol levels, ease inflammation, stabilize heart rhythm, and prevent cardiovascular disease in other ways. A clean diet reduces or eliminates "bad" fats—saturated and trans fats—but includes healthful amounts of good fats.

  The soluble fiber found in beans, oats, flaxseed, and oat bran, according to the Mayo Clinic, may also contribute to lowering cholesterol levels.
- **Look younger.** Antioxidants—nutrients that are found abundantly in fresh fruits and vegetables—fight against free radicals that damage cells and cause inflammation, both of which cause the skin to show signs of aging, such as

wrinkles and dark spots. According to WebMD's guide, "Aging Well," and Samantha Cassetty on WebMD, a diet that includes plenty of high-antioxidant foods like fresh berries can reduce or prevent the physical signs of aging, keep your complexion smooth, and contribute to lustrous hair.

Eating refined sugar also compromises your immune system and speeds the physical effects of aging. According to Dr. Frederic Brandt on Prevention.com, sugar speeds the breakdown of collagen and elastin, proteins that keep the skin smooth, elastic, and glowing.

- **Lower your risk for cancer.** According to the American Cancer Society, consuming a diet high in heavily processed foods elevates your risk of cancer. Eating a clean diet rich in whole grains, monounsaturated fats, and fresh fruits and vegetables, however, can significantly lower your cancer risk, by helping you maintain an appropriate weight and by boosting your intake of healthful phytonutrients and antioxidants that fight cancer growth.

Clean Eating and Paleo: What's the Difference?

Both clean eating and Paleo diets have become increasingly popular recently, and there are many similarities between the two. The two diet plans focus on eliminating processed foods, artificial ingredients, added sugars, and alcohol. Both also encourage choosing whole foods and eating more fresh fruits and vegetables.

So what *is* the difference? Well, to start with, the Paleo diet seeks to re-create the diet of our ancestors—the diet humans ate when we lived as hunter-gatherers before we developed agricultural practices. As a result, the Paleo diet advocates not just eliminating foods with artificial ingredients and refined sugars or grains, but eating only the types of foods that would have been available to our prehistoric ancestors: whole fruits, vegetables, raw nuts and seeds, and meat. Favored by athletes who thrive on a high-protein, low-carb regimen, the Paleo diet eschews cultivated grains and beans and legumes, as well as dairy products.

The clean eating diet, on the other hand, is less restrictive. It seeks to replace refined and processed foods with whole, natural foods, but it does allow whole grains, dairy products, and beans and legumes. Clean eating tends to appeal more to those who don't like to cook or eat meat as often as is required by the Paleo diet.

- **Be happier.** Some of the nutrients from your diet—like vitamins B_6, B_{12}, and folate—help in the production of neurotransmitters, like dopamine, one of the brain chemicals responsible for feelings of pleasure. According to the Mayo Clinic, deficiencies in these nutrients can lead to depression or other mood disorders. Eating a diet rich in healthful sources of these foods—nuts, seeds, avocados, lean meats, and fish—can contribute to good mental health.

Six Principles of Clean Eating

The premise underlying clean eating is to consume a balanced diet made up of wholesome, natural foods. The following principles are based on current research in nutrition and echo the recommendations made by public health organizations to optimize your health by eating a healthful balance of complex carbohydrates, good fats, and lean proteins.

1. **Choose whole foods over packaged foods.** Instead of foods that come in boxes, bags, cans, or packages with long lists of ingredients, choose unprocessed, single-ingredient foods such as fresh fruits and vegetables and whole grains.

2. **Choose foods in the closest form possible to how they are found in nature.** While you may not always be able to choose whole, unrefined foods, strive to choose foods made from whole grains and sweetened with unrefined sweeteners such as honey, maple syrup, or dehydrated cane juice over foods made with refined grain flours and sugars.

3. **Eat balanced meals that include protein along with carbohydrates and healthful fats.** Every meal should include protein along with carbohydrates and fats. Protein helps build muscle and curb your appetite, allowing you to feel full and satisfied longer, which is especially beneficial if you are trying to lose weight.

4. **Avoid saturated or trans fats, excess salt, and refined sugar.** Whole foods are naturally low in fat, sugar, and salt, so cutting out processed foods makes this principle easier to follow than you might think.

5. **Eat several small meals throughout the day.** Whether you eat six mini meals or three meals and one or two healthful snacks each day, eating every few hours keeps you from getting too hungry and then binging or overeating. It also stabilizes your blood sugar so your energy doesn't crash midway through the day.

6. **Drink plenty of water.** At least 8 glasses per day. Choose water over high-calorie beverages—specialty coffee drinks, sodas, juices, alcoholic beverages, and the like—that are low in nutrients and can add at least 500 extra calories to your daily diet. If you need a break from plain water, try sparkling mineral water, spike it with a squeeze of lemon or lime juice, or choose unsweetened herbal tea.

Forget Calories, Remember Portions

Generally speaking, clean eating doesn't encourage counting calories. If you are eating only clean foods, the thinking goes, you aren't at risk for loading up on the kinds of empty calories you get in, say, donuts or cookies, and therefore eating the proper number of calories should happen naturally. Moreover, most clean foods are low in calories, and those that are higher in calories—like olive oil and avocados—contain good fats instead of saturated or trans fats. There's a popular saying: "Eating clean makes you lean."

The stance against calorie counting in the clean eating plan comes from the idea that if you are eating only healthful, whole foods that are nutrient dense and you are paying attention to your body's signals of hunger and satiety, then you should be able to tell intuitively when you've eaten enough. But there's no rule against calorie counting, and some people may feel the need to count calories, at least in the beginning, especially those who are trying to lose weight or making a significant change from an unhealthy way of eating to eating clean. To this end, each recipe in this book contains nutritional information, including calorie counts. By keeping track of the calories in your meals, you can gain an understanding of how many calories different foods have, how much your body needs in order to feel satisfied, and, equally important, what it feels like when you've overdone it.

> **What Does a Serving Look Like?**
>
> Many food guides recommend using your eyes to get a sense of what a proper serving size is. These guides usually compare servings to objects like baseballs, tennis balls, dice, or decks of cards. A simpler way to eyeball serving sizes is to use your hand as a comparative tool. You always have it with you, so there's less chance of miscalculating. Here's a key:
>
> 1 serving of whole grains = your cupped palm (½ cup)
> 1 serving of vegetables = your fist or both palms cupped together (1 cup)
> 1 serving of lean protein = the flat palm of your hand (3 ounces)
> 1 serving of fat = the top half of your thumb (1 teaspoon)
> 1 serving of cheese = your thumb (1 ounce)
> 1 serving of nuts or seeds = ½ of your cupped palm (¼ cup)

Whether or not you choose to count calories, you'll want to keep portion sizes and serving numbers of food types in mind when planning your meals in order to ensure that you are not overeating and that you are getting the right mix of nutrients. Most experts recommend a diet that is 40 to 50 percent carbohydrates, 25 to 35 percent protein, and 20 to 30 percent fat. This means that each day, you should eat roughly six to ten servings of complex carbohydrates, five to six servings of lean protein, and two to three servings of heart-healthy fats.

Foods to Enjoy

You may be worried that once you cut out all the packaged, processed, and refined foods from your diet, you'll be left with an alarmingly short list of allowable foods. More than likely, though, once you start eating clean and exploring all that the world of whole, natural foods has to offer, you'll be pleasantly surprised at the variety of delicious, nutritious, and satisfying foods available to you.

Seasonal and Local

Choosing in-season foods increases the likelihood that the food you are eating is very fresh, has been grown locally, and was picked more recently, which means that it likely still contains the bulk of its nutrients. The longer produce sits and the farther it is transported after being harvested, the more nutrients it loses.

Equally important, fresh in-season produce tastes better. Have you ever plucked a perfectly ripe, warm-from-the-sun cherry tomato from the vine and popped it in your mouth? If so, you can probably taste in your mind right now the explosion of sweet-tart tomatoey flavor. The same is true for most produce: Fresh picked, seasonal produce just tastes better.

It also costs a pretty penny to ship blueberries from Chile to the United States in winter, and you pay that cost. In-season, locally grown produce will likely eat up less of your grocery budget, leaving you more to spend on quality meats, grains, and other foods.

Conventional Versus Organic

As you shop for groceries, keep in mind that conventional produce-growing techniques involve the use of chemical pesticides and fertilizers. Conventionally raised meats and conventionally produced dairy products may be treated with antibiotics and artificial growth hormones. In a perfect world, you would choose only organic produce, meat, and dairy. Unfortunately, because of availability and budget concerns, organic foods are not always accessible. In the next chapter, you'll find out which conventional produce and veggies are okay to buy and which organic items should be purchased if possible. If you do choose conventionally grown produce, make sure to wash it thoroughly to get rid of much of the chemical residue. If you choose conventionally raised meat and dairy, look for products that state on the label that the animals are not treated with hormones or antibiotics.

Here are the foods that are encouraged on the clean eating menu:

Fresh Fruits
- apples
- apricots
- bananas
- blackberries
- blueberries
- cherries
- coconut
- grapes
- oranges
- peaches
- pears
- pineapple
- raspberries
- strawberries

Fresh Vegetables
artichokes
asparagus
avocados
beets
bell peppers
broccoli
Brussels sprouts
cabbage
carrots
cauliflower
celery
chard
cucumbers
eggplant
garlic
green beans
kale
leeks
lettuce
onions
parsnips
potatoes
radishes
scallions
snow peas
spinach
sugar snap peas
sweet potatoes
tomatoes
turnips
zucchini

Herbs and Spices
basil
black peppercorns
cayenne pepper
chiles
chili powder
cilantro
cinnamon
cloves
cumin
ginger
mustard
nutmeg
oregano
parsley
rosemary
sage
tarragon
thyme
turmeric

Whole Grains
amaranth
barley
brown rice
bulgur
corn
farro
millet
oats
quinoa
spelt
wheat berries

Nuts and Seeds
(including all-natural, nothing-added nut butters and seed butters)
almonds
cashews
chia seeds
flaxseed
hazelnuts
macadamia nuts
peanuts
pecans
pine nuts
pumpkin seeds (pepitas)
sunflower seeds
walnuts

Legumes
black beans
black-eyed peas
butter beans
chickpeas
fava beans
kidney beans
lentils
lima beans
peas
pinto beans
soy beans (edamame)

Lean Proteins
eggs (large)
poultry
fish
shellfish
beef
pork
lamb

Dairy Products
milk
yogurt
cheeses that are naturally low in fat, such as:
  cottage cheese
  feta cheese
  goat cheese
  fresh mozzarella, ricotta
  whipped cream cheese

Healthful Fats
almond oil
avocado oil
avocados
coconut oil
olive oil
olives
safflower oil
sunflower oil
walnut oil

Milk Substitutes
(check labels for no additives)
almond milk
cashew milk
coconut milk
hemp milk
soy milk

Treats and Unrefined Sweeteners
(in limited quantities)
coconut sugar
dark chocolate
dehydrated cane sugar
honey
maple syrup

Unsweetened, Nonalcoholic Beverages
coffee
tea (iced or hot black, or herbal tea)
water and sparkling water (without additives)

Foods to Avoid

While the clean diet is flexible, certain foods should not be eaten. The good news is that once you get used to your clean eating diet, those foods likely won't appeal to you anymore.

Packaged Foods

The largest category of foods to avoid includes any food that comes in a package with a lengthy list of often unrecognizable ingredients, including preservatives, artificial colors, artificial and "natural" flavors, stabilizers, emulsifiers, and thickeners.

Refined Sweeteners

Refined sweeteners, like white sugar and high-fructose corn syrup, are a no-no on the clean eating plan, for good reason. They deliver no nutritional value, are loaded with empty calories, and contribute to inflammation that causes a host of ailments from obesity and diabetes to heart disease, high blood pressure, arthritis pain, and premature aging.

Refined Grains

When grain is refined, it goes through a process in which the whole grain is stripped of its bran, germ, and endosperm. While this makes for fluffy flours that produce delicate cakes and delightful sandwich breads, it also strips the grains of most of their nutritional value—the fiber, vitamins, and minerals your body needs to thrive. Stay away from highly refined white flour (often listed as "wheat flour"), white rice flour, and other highly refined grain flours, and you'll reduce symptoms of high blood sugar, food cravings, inflammation, and fatigue.

Trans Fat and Saturated Fat

The "bad" fats include saturated fats and trans fats. Trans fats are created when oils are hydrogenated to increase their shelf life or improve the texture or mouthfeel of processed or packaged foods.

Saturated fat occurs naturally in animal products, including meat and dairy products. Too much saturated fat increases your risk of a lengthy list of diseases such as obesity, heart disease, and certain types of cancer. A limited amount of saturated fat from natural sources is okay on the clean eating plan, but only in very small quantities.

Other Foods to Avoid

- High-calorie beverages: bottled fruit juices, alcoholic beverages, sweetened coffee drinks, energy drinks, sodas
- Hydrogenated fats: margarine, processed foods that contain hydrogenated or partially hydrogenated oil

- Food additives: colors, flavors, preservatives, thickeners, emulsifiers, stabilizers, artificial sweeteners.
- Dairy products high in saturated fat: hard cheeses, butter, cream
- Fried foods
- Frozen or packaged processed foods
- Fatty meats: cured bacon or other cured meats that contain nitrates and nitrites, and packaged sausage, hot dogs, salami and other deli meats, and hamburgers
- Baked goods made with refined flours: breads, brownies, cakes, cookies, rolls, pastries, rolls
- Packaged conventional pasta
- White rice
- Packaged processed breakfast cereals
- Packaged snack foods: potato chips, pretzels, crackers
- Sweets: store-bought candy, ice cream
- Soybean oil, canola oil, palm oil, palm kernel oil, and vegetable oil
- Farmed fish like salmon and tilapia
- Meats and dairy products that come from animals treated with antibiotics or growth hormones
- Coffee creamers and sweetened nondairy milk

Top Seven FAQs About Clean Eating

1. **I don't have a lot of time to cook. Will I still be able to adopt the clean eating plan?** Yes. There are many clean foods that don't require much preparation or extensive cooking to be delicious. Fresh, raw fruits, vegetables, nuts, and seeds are great bases for both meals and snacks. Add cooked beans and simply prepared lean proteins, and you're good to go. While eating clean does require more effort and more time in the kitchen than grabbing takeout or microwaving a frozen meal, once you get into the swing of it, you'll find there are many ways to maximize your efforts so that you can eat healthful meals even on busy weekdays.

2. **Is it possible to eat clean as a vegetarian or vegan?** Absolutely. Many, even most, clean foods are naturally meat-free. Beans, nuts, seeds, and whole grains can easily provide all of the protein you need. If you're an ovo-lacto vegetarian, you can also enjoy eggs and certain dairy products. And vegans will find plenty of nutritious foods on the clean eating diet.

3. **How can I possibly cook without refined flour?** Whole-grain flours are considered "clean" and can often be used in place of refined wheat flour. These include whole-wheat, oat, amaranth, teff, barley, quinoa, and brown rice flours, among others. There are also many grain-free flours available that can be substituted for conventional grain-based flours with a bit of recipe tweaking, including coconut flour, almond flour, and chickpea flour. These flours are made from fruits, nuts, or legumes, and can be used in recipes that call for flour to dredge meats or thicken sauces. Many of the recipes in this book demonstrate how these flours can be used to replace grain flours in baking and other applications.

4. **Can I eat as much fruit and vegetables as I want?** Fresh fruit is allowed on the clean eating diet, but do limit your intake to two or three servings per day since fruit does contain quite a bit of sugar. Nonstarchy vegetables (like leafy greens, broccoli, Brussels sprouts, cauliflower) are low in calories and high in nutrients, so feel free to eat as much as you like for breakfast, lunch, dinner, and in between. Starchy vegetables, such as corn, peas, potatoes, and sweet potatoes, on the other hand, are high in calories,

so they should be eaten in limited quantities. Limit yourself to two or three servings of starchy vegetables per day.

5. **I thought canola oil was healthful. Why is it on the "Foods to Avoid" list?** Canola oil has been marketed as a lower-cost alternative to olive oil. Like olive oil, it is low in saturated fat and high in monounsaturated fat. But unlike olive oil, canola oil is a newly developed food product that is made from a genetically engineered plant (the rapeseed plant). Very few studies have been done on the healthfulness of canola oil. Furthermore, the best olive oils are produced by cold-pressing olives, which preserves the stability and nutritional qualities of the oil, and then bottling the oil. Canola oil, on the other hand, is produced through a combination of high-temperature pressing, which can break down the oil's heart-healthy fats, and the use of a chemical solvent, and then it is put through an intense high-temperature refining process that can further break down the heart-healthy fats, introduce trans fats, and leave additional chemical residue. Do yourself a favor and stick to "clean" oils like almond, coconut, olive, safflower, and sunflower oil.

6. **I'm on a tight budget. How can I eat clean without breaking the bank?** Clean eating can seem expensive at first because of its focus on organic, fresh, and all-natural foods, but this book is designed to help maximize your grocery budget by providing a detailed four-week meal plan. By planning ahead, buying and cooking in bulk when possible, and utilizing leftovers for future meals, you can eat well without spending a lot. Other tricks for keeping grocery costs down include eliminating takeout, shopping for bargains, buying local and seasonal produce, buying organic meats frozen in bulk, and forgoing expensive organic produce for items on the Environmental Working Group's "Clean Fifteen" list (see page 21)—conventionally grown fruits and vegetables that have very low chemical residue levels.

7. **I know they say breakfast is the most important meal of the day, but I'm always in a rush. Can I skip it?** Absolutely not. For one thing, breakfast gives you the energy to begin your day. And it has numerous health benefits such as kick-starting your metabolism, which burns calories and helps you maintain an appropriate weight and improved mental clarity and performance. According to WebMD and Eatright.org, children who skip breakfast perform worse in the classroom and have a harder time with concentration, problem-solving skills, and eye-hand coordination. It's likely that a missed breakfast has the same effect on adults. If you are pressed for time in the mornings, whip up a frittata and cut it into wedges, make a batch of mini egg muffins, or bake homemade power bars and wrap them for easy grab-and-go breakfasts.

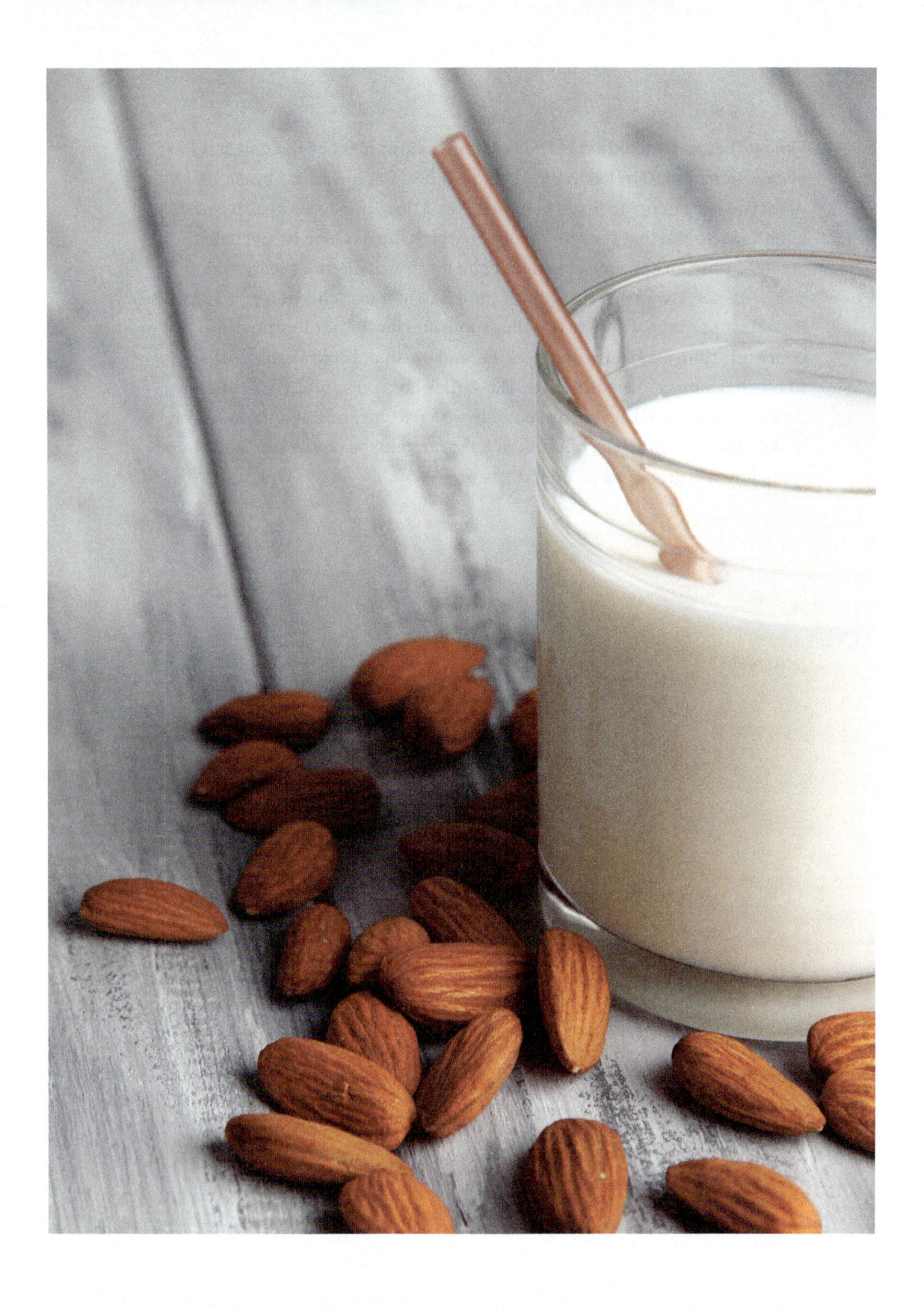

How to Use the Meal Plan

Making the change to clean eating can seem daunting at first. This book provides a detailed four-week meal plan that can help ease you into the process by taking the guesswork out of the daily question, "What's for dinner (or breakfast, or lunch)?" The meal plan covers breakfast, lunch, dinner, and dessert for each day plus snack suggestions, so you'll know what to eat for every meal and snack of every day.

Following a set meal plan will also help you save time and money and reduce waste. That's because the meal plan has been designed to use up leftovers and utilize the same ingredients in multiple ways throughout the week.

In the following chapters, you will find all the tools you need to get started on your clean eating plan. At the end of the four weeks, choosing fresh, whole foods over processed foods with lots of additives will feel completely natural to you. You will have developed habits that can turn you into a clean eater for life.

Getting the Most out of Your Meal Plan

The four-week meal plan provides 28 days of preplanned meals divided by week. Each week's plan begins with a snapshot of the week's meals so you can get a sense of what's coming up. Also, each week includes a list of pantry items you'll use (including an indication of how much you'll need of each ingredient so that you can check to see if you've got enough), a convenient grocery shopping list you can take to the market, and tips for what and how to prep ahead for some of the meals.

The meal plan details specific meals (with recipes included in the recipe section of the book) for each day, for breakfast, lunch, and dinner. For snacks, at the beginning of each week, you can choose from a list of snack suggestions—including nine ready-made snacks and three make-ahead snack suggestions (with recipes included in the recipe section). To stave off hunger, you should be sure to eat one or two snacks from the list each day.

To help you get the most out of your time spent in the kitchen—and out of your food budget—the meal plan includes recipes that have been created specifically to generate leftovers that are then used in future meals. For instance, Sunday's roasted chicken dinner becomes Chicken Enchiladas Verdes with Goat Cheese for dinner on Tuesday as well as Spinach Salad with Chicken and Sun-Dried Tomato and Basil Vinaigrette for Wednesday's lunch.

Because sauces, dressings, condiments, and some other refrigerator and pantry staples can be especially troublesome for clean eaters, we've included recipes for many of these. These recipes are used in the meal plans, and once you've made them for one dish, you'll have leftovers to use in future dishes.

Most of the recipes in the book are designed to make four servings (and more, for certain dishes like baked goods and snacks). If you're cooking for a family of four, you'll be able to use most of the recipes as is. If you are cooking for more people, most recipes are easily doubled. If you are cooking for fewer people, most recipes can be halved, or in many cases you can cook the full amount and store leftovers in the refrigerator or freezer for future meals.

Learn to Read Food Labels

Food labels are one of your best sources of information about that food item. Of course, the "cleanest" foods are those that don't come with labels—organic fresh fruits, vegetables, and meats—but for most of us, packaged foods of some sort are a necessary evil because they are convenient and widely accessible. If you plan to buy any packaged foods—whether it's a box of cookies or a bag of organic spelt flour—the label will tell you what is in the food before you put it in your body.

Is Fresh Always Best?

Some days it can be a challenge to eat the recommended amount of fruits and vegetables. And during the winter months, or if you live in an area without much access to fresh produce year-round, it gets that much harder. You may wonder if frozen or canned produce is anywhere near as nutritious as fresh.

The canning process, since it involves processing at high temperatures, does in fact deplete most foods of many of their nutrients. Furthermore, most canned goods are full of additives and excess sodium. There are a couple of exceptions, notably tomatoes and pumpkin, which retain their nutrients even through the canning process. Do look for canned versions without salt, sugar, or other additives, though. It is also recommended that you choose tomatoes packaged in boxes rather than cans to avoid exposure to BPA (bisphenol-A). Because of tomatoes' natural acidity, canned tomatoes are among the foods most likely to contain BPA leached from the can's lining. Whenever possible, choose tomatoes packaged in boxes rather than in cans to avoid this risk. There are some brands of canned organic tomatoes listed as BPA-free (such as Amy's, Eden Foods, Muir Glen, Trader Joe's, Whole Foods), but you may want to do your own research on the issue of BPA and canned foods on the Internet.

When it comes to frozen produce, however, the answer is much different. In many cases, frozen produce is actually more nutritious than its fresh counterpart in the supermarket, according to Gene Lester and Rachael Moeller Gorman on eatingwell.com. For one thing, produce destined for freezing is picked at the peak of ripeness, which is when it is the most full of nutrients. Flash-freezing them suspends them in this nutrient-dense state. Fresh produce destined for wide distribution, on the other hand, is often picked underripe—when fruits and vegetables haven't yet developed the full spectrum of nutrients—to prevent spoiling in transit. The nutrient content also may be degraded during distribution as the produce is exposed to variations in light and temperature.

The best advice is to buy in-season produce when it is fresh and ripe, but when buying out-of-season produce, frozen versions are probably the way to go.

Ingredients List

Check for any ingredients you don't recognize or can't pronounce. Artificial colors, flavors, preservatives, stabilizers, emulsifiers, thickeners, and other additives should be avoided whenever possible. Choose packaged foods with short ingredient lists that include only natural ingredients that you recognize and understand.

Next, examine the list for refined grains or sweeteners. These include white flour (may be listed as "wheat flour") or any other highly processed flour. Allowable grain flours include 100 percent whole wheat, spelt, teff, amaranth, quinoa, and others made exclusively from whole grains.

Refined sugars, including white sugar (often listed simply as "sugar"), brown sugar, corn syrup or corn sweetener, barley malt, beet sugar, cane juice, and palm sugar, are to be avoided. Unrefined sweeteners like honey, maple syrup, and coconut sugar are allowed on the clean eating plan in limited quantities.

Nutrition Facts

This portion of the label is also valuable. Although counting calories isn't necessary on the clean eating plan, it's still important to pay attention to serving sizes and keep your portions within the recommended range for your size, age, and gender. You'll find the serving size listed, along with the number of calories per serving, micrograms of cholesterol, and grams of fat (overall, and trans and saturated fats), protein, and fiber.

Look at the overall fat content, as well as the amount of saturated or trans fat in the food. While it's a good idea to limit excess fat in your diet, the fats you really want to avoid are cholesterol-raising saturated and trans fats. Saturated fat should be consumed in very limited quantities, while trans fat—created through an industrial process designed to make liquid vegetable oils solid at room temperature and increase a food's shelf life—should be avoided altogether.

The Dirty Dozen and The Clean Fifteen

THE DIRTY DOZEN

Apple
Bell pepper
Celery
Cherry tomato
Cucumber
Grape
Nectarine
   (imported)
Peach
Potato
Snap pea
   (imported)
Spinach
Strawberry

Each year, Environmental Working Group, an environmental organization based in the United States, publishes a list they call the "Dirty Dozen." These are the fruits and vegetables that, when conventionally grown using chemical pesticides and fertilizers, carry the highest residues. If organically grown isn't an option for you, simply avoid these fruits and vegetables altogether. The list is updated each year, but this is the most recent list (2014).

Similarly, the Environmental Working Group publishes a list of "The Clean Fifteen," fruits and vegetables that, even when conventionally grown, contain very low levels of chemical pesticide or fertilizer residue. These items are acceptable for purchasing conventionally grown.

You might want to snap a photo of these two lists and keep them on your phone to reference while shopping. Or you can download the Environmental Working Group's app to your phone or tablet (visit www.ewg.org).

THE CLEAN FIFTEEN

Asparagus
Avocado
Cabbage
Cantaloupe
Corn
Eggplant
Grapefruit
Kiwi
Mango
Mushroom
Onions
Papaya
Pineapple
Sweet peas
   (frozen)
Sweet potato

Shopping Tips

Clean eating is about making a conscious effort each and every time you eat to choose the most healthful foods possible. The optimum place to make those choices is in the market when you are stocking up on foods for the week, not when you've just arrived home from work, starving, at 6:30 p.m. Make good choices in the supermarket, and you'll continue to make good choices from your refrigerator and pantry all week long.

Stock Your Pantry

Starting out on a clean eating diet means you'll need to sort through your pantry and dispose of any offending foods or ingredients, such as cookies, crackers, or other snack foods that contain artificial ingredients, refined flour, or refined sugar. You'll also want to toss your bags of refined flour and sugar, as well as any other ingredients that aren't allowed on the plan. Next you'll want to restock your pantry with the ingredients needed for making the recipes in this book and other clean recipes.

The following lists include all the pantry items you'll need to make all of the recipes in this book. Be sure to check food labels before purchasing, to make sure the versions of these items you buy are clean.

Oils

clean cooking oil, such as grapeseed
coconut oil
olive oil
sesame oil

Herbs and Spices

black peppercorns
cayenne pepper
chili powder
cinnamon (ground)
cumin (ground)
curry powder
dill (dried)
garlic
onions
oregano (dried)
sea salt or kosher salt
smoked paprika
turmeric (ground)
thai red curry paste
wasabi powder

Sweeteners

coconut sugar
honey
maple syrup

A Closer Look at Coconut Oil

In the health food world, coconut oil is currently the big thing. Not too long ago, the flavorful oil was thought to be virtual poison since it's so high in saturated fat, but the tides have turned. Coconut oil is now held up by many, including Dr. Pina LoGiudice, as the ultimate health food cure-all. There have been reports that it can boost immune function, cure thyroid disease and heart disease, help with weight loss, boost metabolism, prevent obesity, and lower the risk of cancer. More research is needed to substantiate each of these claims, but according to the Center for Science in the Public Interest, its high concentration of medium-chain triglycerides (MCTs) are metabolized by the body differently than the long-chain triglycerides found in most cooking oils. These MCTs are transported directly from the digestive tract to the liver, where they are burned for quick energy rather than being deposited into the body's fat tissues. This provides a slight, but possibly significant, boost to metabolism.

While coconut oil may or may not be the new wonder food cure-all, many health-conscious people choose to cook with it simply because it is a very stable oil that is solid at room temperature; doesn't oxidize, spoil, or turn rancid easily; has a high smoke point; and unlike some other cooking oils, doesn't produce harmful chemicals when used over high heat. Look for virgin or extra-virgin, cold-pressed coconut oil, which you can find in natural food stores, health food stores, and many supermarkets.

Flours and Grains

Arborio rice
arrowroot starch
almond flour
brown rice
coconut flour
ground flaxseed
oat flour
old-fashioned rolled oats
quinoa
whole-wheat flour
whole-wheat pasta

Condiments

apple cider vinegar
balsamic vinegar
chili paste (optional)
Dijon mustard
mirin (Japanese sweet rice wine)
rice vinegar
sherry vinegar
soy sauce (low-sodium)
white wine vinegar

Dried Fruit, Nuts, Nut and Seed Butters
almonds (whole, roasted, unsalted, sliced)
cashews
coconut (shredded, unsweetened)
cranberries (dried, unsweetened)
dates (pitted)
peanut butter (all-natural)
pecans
pineapple (dried)
raisins
sesame seeds
tahini
walnuts

Beans and Legumes
black beans (canned)
cannellini beans (canned)
chickpeas (canned)
red lentils (dried)

Frozen Produce
blueberries
corn kernels
green beans
peas
soy beans (edamame)
spinach
strawberries

Other
baking powder
baking soda
broth (canned; chicken, beef, vegetable)
cocoa powder (unsweetened)
coconut milk (canned)
green chiles (canned, diced)
nutritional yeast
pineapple chunks (canned)
roasted red bell peppers (jarred, in water)
tomatoes (both crushed and diced, canned or packaged in boxes)
tomato paste
sun-dried tomatoes packed in oil
vanilla extract
yeast (quick-rising)

Essential Tools and Equipment

Clean eating may require you to do more cooking than you're used to, but you don't need a lot of fancy equipment. And you likely have most of the equipment already. There are just a couple of kitchen tools—a food processor and a blender—that are essential for some of the recipes in the book.

In addition, an electric mixer (a hand mixer or a stand mixer) is useful for making some of the baked goods but is not necessary.

A waffle iron is recommended for the Protein-Packed Freezer Waffles (page 66), but if you don't have one, you can use the batter to make pancakes instead.

If you choose to make Homemade Almond Milk (page 225), a fine-mesh nut milk bag or a square of cheesecloth makes the job easier.

Healthful Cooking Methods

The most healthful cooking methods are those that maintain a food's inherent nutritional value without adding excess fat (or any other undesirables like sugar, salt, or even carcinogens from char grilling, for that matter). There are many different ways to cook that keep food's nutrients intact and allow you to create healthful dishes. It's an added bonus that some of these cooking methods are also the simplest.

Baking and Roasting

Baking is not just for breads, cookies, and cakes. You can also bake meats and vegetables, and this method deepens and intensifies flavors without adding fat. All you need is a pan and a hot oven. You can coat meats and vegetables with herbs and spices before baking to infuse them with flavor, but adding a bit of fat will help the seasonings stick and the flavors permeate.

Roasting, similar to baking, is done at a higher temperature, which causes the natural sugars in the food to caramelize, giving the finished dish a deep, complex flavor. For best results, coat the food with a smidgen of healthful fat before roasting. Roasting can be done with meat, seafood, fish, or vegetables.

Braising, Poaching, Steaming, and Boiling

Braising is a method of cooking foods—usually tougher cuts of meat, but vegetables and other foods can also be braised—slowly in simmering liquid. Meats generally should be seared in a hot pan first to brown the outside and seal in the juices, and then cooked slowly in a small quantity of simmering liquid (such as broth, stock, or water) with whatever herbs and spices you would like to add.

Poaching is similar to braising in that food is cooked in a simmering liquid. Generally done faster and at a higher temperature than braising, poaching is used for more delicate foods like eggs and fish.

One of the simplest cooking techniques is steaming food in a perforated basket suspended above simmering liquid. If you use a flavorful liquid or add seasonings to the water, you'll flavor the food as it cooks without any added fat. Boiling is when you submerge food in boiling water and cook it quickly. While it can be done without adding any extra fat, many of the food's nutrients may leach out into the boiling water and get poured down the drain.

Sautéing and Stir-Frying

Sautéing involves cooking usually small pieces of food at medium-high temperature and moving the pieces around quickly. Sautéing is best done with a small amount of added fat, but if you use a good nonstick pan, you won't need much. Stir-frying is similar to sautéing but is done at very high heat. As with sautéing, just a little bit of fat is all you need if you use a good nonstick pan or wok.

Healthful Grilling

Grilling—cooking meat over the heat of hot coals or on a gas grill—is a mixed bag when it comes to health. One of the standard diet mantras is to choose grilled foods over fried. And it is good advice in that a grilled chicken breast, for instance, will have much less fat than fried chicken. But not all grilling is healthy. When fat from meat drips onto the grill and flames and smoke leap up and lick the food being grilled, a couple of cancer-causing compounds—polycyclic aromatic hydrocarbons (PAHs) and heterocyclic amines (HCAs)—are created and deposited onto the food.

The good news, though, is that PAHs and HCAs don't form when grilling fruits or veggies, so you can grill those to your heart's content. Grilling lean meats and fish, too, is safer since less fat dripping on the grill means less chance of those nasty compounds forming. Choose lean cuts, trim visible fat, and remove skin from poultry before grilling, and you'll cut the risk significantly.

Microwaving

There is a lot of debate about whether microwave cooking is good or bad for you. On the one hand, according to the Harvard School of Public Health, because microwaving cooks food quickly, it may help the food retain more nutrients than other longer cooking methods like steaming, poaching, or boiling. On the other hand, microwaving in non-microwave-safe containers can cause food to become infused with dangerous chemicals. The bottom line is that microwaving is safe and healthful provided you cook food for only as much time as it needs to cook through and always use microwave-safe containers made of glass or ceramic (check the bottom of the container for use in the microwave).

10 Tips to Make Clean Eating Work for You

Eating clean will leave you feeling healthy and full of vitality. The trade-off is that clean eating requires you to prep and cook most of your meals yourself. Here are a few tips to make the transition a bit easier.

1. **Focus on the healthful, delicious foods you are adding to your diet, not on what you are being deprived of.** It's easy to fall into a feeling of deprivation when you first start a clean eating diet, since you may have to give up foods you enjoy. But you will be adding foods that are not just more nutritious, but also delicious. It may be difficult at first, but soon you'll start to love the new foods as much as the old. And if you're like most people, unhealthful foods will lose their appeal after an extended period of clean eating.

2. **Buy organic meats in bulk.** To keep costs down and ensure that you always have healthful proteins on hand for meals, look for bargains on organic meats and then stock up. Split whatever you don't intend to use the next day or two into meal-size portions, wrap them well, and freeze them for later use. Be sure to label and date the packages. Meat can be kept frozen without compromising quality for three months or longer.

3. **Buy seasonal produce.** In-season, locally grown produce is less expensive than out-of-season produce or fruits and vegetables that have been shipped in from far away. Look for good deals and then stock up. Fresh berries and other fruits can be frozen, as can hearty vegetables like corn, broccoli, or cauliflower.

4. **Cook in bulk.** If you're making a pot of soup or chili, a lasagna or enchiladas, or another freezer-friendly meal, double the recipe and then freeze the extra in meal-size portions so you'll have meals on hand that only need to be defrosted.

5. **Prep once, cook twice.** Eating clean will likely require you to spend more time in the kitchen than you're used to. Minimize your time in the kitchen by doubling up on preparation tasks like chopping vegetables. For instance, if you are chopping an onion for a dish tonight, why not chop two onions and bag one and save it for tomorrow night's dinner? This will make your time in the kitchen much more efficient.

6. **Keep healthful snacks on hand at all times.** Nuts, seeds, dried fruits, and homemade granola make great snacks. Tuck them in your purse, your car, and your desk drawer at work, so you'll always have a clean snack available when hunger strikes.

7. **Eat protein at every meal.** It's easy to fill up on carbohydrates, but protein will satisfy your hunger in fewer calories, and that satisfied feeling will last longer. Choose lean proteins, like white-meat fish or chicken, or beans to keep calories and saturated fats in check.

8. **Eat healthful fats at every meal.** Healthful fats are an essential part of a healthful diet because they help the body absorb important nutrients and they provide a feeling of satiety. Fat also slows the body's absorption of sugars, helping stabilize blood sugar. Be sure to include healthful fats—like from avocados, nuts, seeds, and healthful oils like olive or coconut—in every meal and snack.

9. **Spice it up.** Boredom is the enemy of any healthful eating plan. Happily, herbs and spices are clean foods and can be used in myriad ways to add flavor and interest to your meals. Stock your spice cabinet well and experiment with different flavor combinations to keep mealtime interesting.

10. **Eat three meals and one or two snacks each day.** Letting yourself get too hungry is a recipe for diet disaster. Think about it. If you're starving, are you going to choose to go home and cook yourself a healthful, clean meal or will you cave to your hunger and pop into the nearest fast-food restaurant for a quick meal? Stave off hunger by eating a healthful meal or snack every few hours, and it will be much easier to stick to healthful choices all day long.

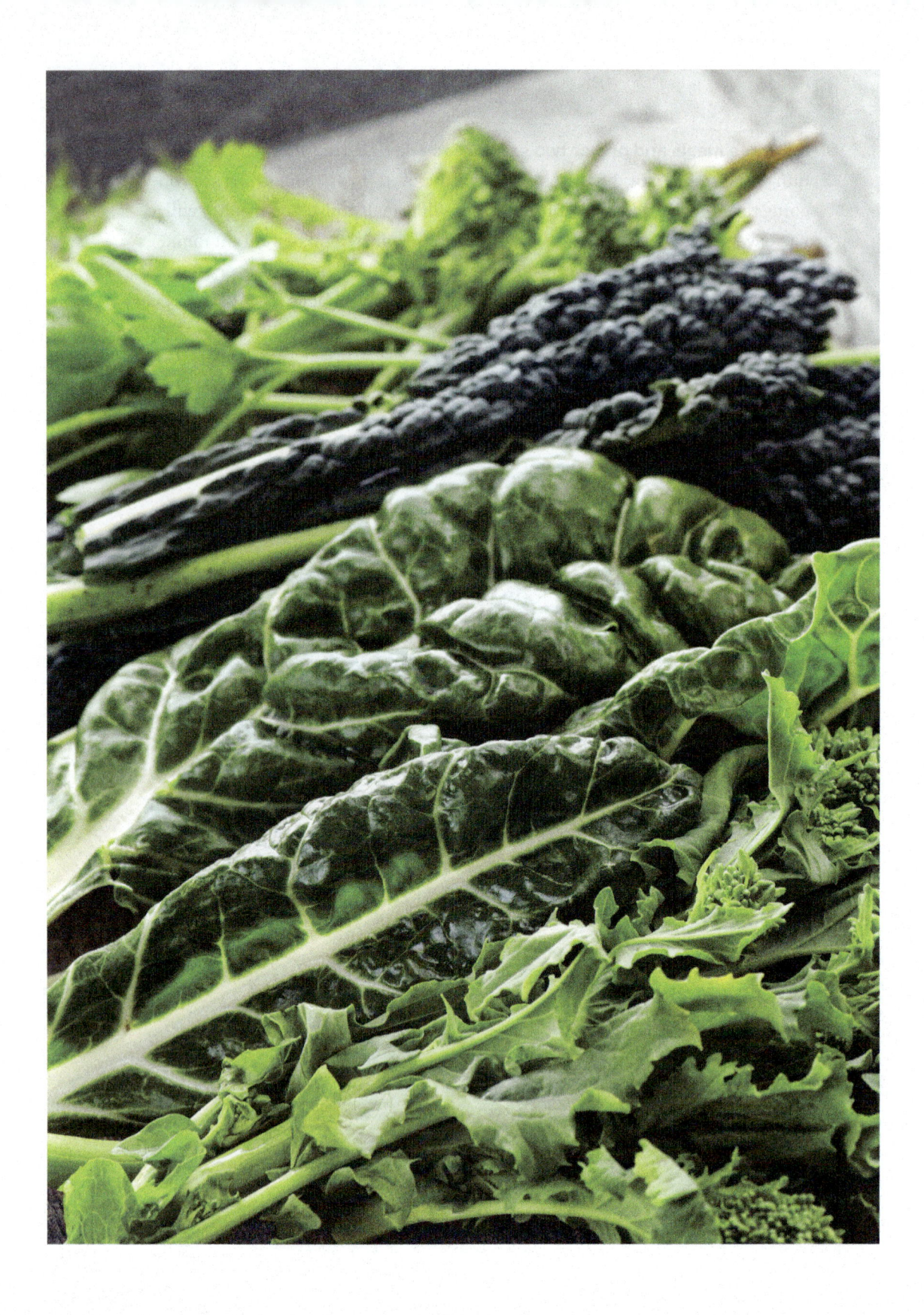

3

Week-by-Week Clean Eating Meal Plans

Your commitment to clean eating begins!

In this chapter, you'll find weekly menus, pantry and shopping lists, and prep-ahead recommendations to reduce the amount of time you spend in the kitchen on weeknights. The menus cover three meals for each day—breakfast, lunch, dinner—and dessert, and offer a list of snacks that you can choose from. Be sure to enjoy one or two snacks between meals each day to avoid getting so hungry that you're tempted to make bad choices.

Enjoying meals is an important part of living life to its fullest, so give yourself the time and space to adjust to this new way of eating.

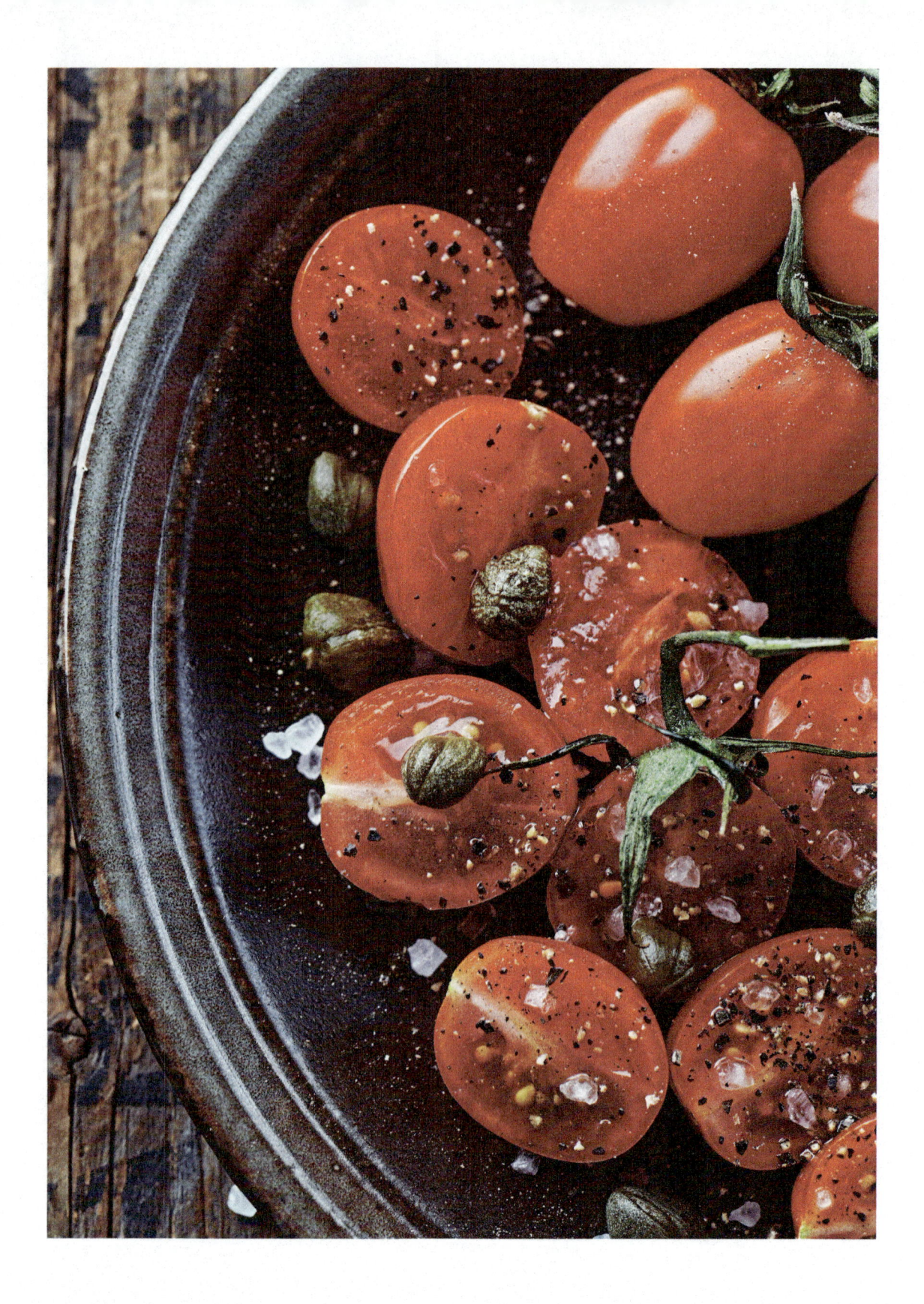

Week One

Be prepared for this to be a challenging week since you'll be just getting used to eating clean. As you learned in Chapter One, two things that often throw off those who are new to the clean eating lifestyle are:

- The cost of buying pantry items and fresh foods
- The time it takes to cook meals, as opposed to ordering in or microwaving

This first week of the meal plan, you will go on a shopping trip, and it will be the biggest you make since you'll be stocking up on staples that you'll often use going forward. Bringing your kitchen up to speed in this way may seem like a large investment, in both money and storage space, but you'll have on hand the clean cooking oils, whole-grain and grain-free flours, natural sweeteners, and clean condiments, stocks, and seasonings you need for cooking all the recipes in this book—and even to create your own original dishes on the fly. Remember, the items for your pantry, cupboard, and even freezer are items that will last you beyond this week, and most of them beyond the four weeks of the meal plan. They'll be regulars in your cooking rotation.

Once you've bought all of the ingredients, it's time to get cooking. There's a learning curve with cooking, and if you're new to the kitchen, there's no getting around the fact that it'll take you longer to chop onions this week than it will next week, and the following week. With practice, you'll decrease the time needed for basic preparation, and cooking will become easier and easier.

Week One Menu at a Glance

Day One
BREAKFAST Scrambled Egg, Goat Cheese, and Cherry Tomato Pita Sandwich
LUNCH Spicy Southwestern Corn and Bean Salad
DINNER Roasted Chicken and Vegetables
DESSERT Banana Chocolate Tart

Day Two
BREAKFAST Homemade Cinnamon Granola
LUNCH Smoky Red Lentil Soup with Greens
DINNER Chicken Enchiladas Verdes with Goat Cheese (use leftover Roasted Chicken from Day One)
DESSERT Rich Chocolate Fudge

Day Three
BREAKFAST Protein-Packed Freezer Waffles (or Pancakes)
LUNCH Spinach Salad with Chicken and Sun-Dried Tomato and Basil Vinaigrette (use leftover Roasted Chicken from Day One)
DINNER Sesame-Soy Marinated Flank Steak with Wasabi-Spiked Cauliflower Purée
DESSERT Molten Chocolate Cakes

Day Four
BREAKFAST Poached Eggs in Spicy Tomato Sauce
LUNCH Quinoa Salad with Cannellini Beans, Tomatoes, and Lemon Vinaigrette
DINNER Grilled Shrimp Tacos with Salsa Verde and Spicy Slaw
DESSERT Banana Maple Nut "Ice Cream"

Day Five

BREAKFAST Ginger Berry Smoothie
LUNCH Curried Chicken Salad Lettuce Wraps with Homemade Mayonnaise
DINNER Goat Cheese and Spinach–Stuffed Pork Chops
DESSERT Peanut Butter Oatmeal Cookies

Day Six

BREAKFAST Whole-Wheat Blueberry Muffins with Cinnamon-Sugar Topping
LUNCH Brown Rice and Black Bean Salad with Spinach and Lemon Vinaigrette
DINNER Whole-Wheat Pasta with Chickpeas and Spicy Tomato Sauce
DESSERT Mini Cheesecakes in Caramel Sauce

Day Seven

BREAKFAST Whole-Wheat Maple Cinnamon Rolls
LUNCH Mediterranean Chickpea Salad with Red Bell Peppers and Feta Cheese
DINNER Quinoa Fried "Rice" with Flank Steak and Peas (leaves leftover quinoa, steak, and veggies)
DESSERT Berry Crumb Cake

SNACKS (CHOOSE ONE OR TWO EACH DAY)

- Roasted almonds and dried fruit
- Plain yogurt with a drizzle of honey, or maple syrup and a handful of chopped nuts
- Lightly salted edamame
- Celery sticks with all-natural nut butter and dried fruit
- Hummus with veggie sticks
- Hard-boiled egg with salt or spices
- Banana with peanut butter
- Basil leaf wraps with goat cheese and cherry tomatoes
- Homemade Cinnamon Granola* with plain Greek yogurt or fresh fruit
- Peanut Butter Energy Bites*
- Basil Garlic Zucchini Chips*
- Spiced Roasted Chickpeas*

Recipe included in recipe section

From the Pantry

Oils
2 cups coconut oil
¾ cup plus 3 tablespoons olive oil
1 tablespoon plus 1 teaspoon sesame oil

Herbs and Spices
Salt
Black peppercorns
13 garlic cloves
5 medium onions
1 teaspoon cayenne pepper
½ teaspoon chili powder
1 tablespoon curry powder
1 tablespoon plus 2½ teaspoons ground cinnamon
2½ teaspoons ground cumin
1 tablespoon dried oregano
2 teaspoons smoked paprika
1 teaspoon ground turmeric
1 teaspoon wasabi powder

Sweeteners
2¾ cups coconut sugar
½ cup plus ½ teaspoon honey
1 cup plus 1 tablespoon maple syrup

Flours and Grains
2½ cups plus 2 tablespoons almond flour
½ cup ground flaxseed
7⅔ cups old-fashioned rolled oats
2 cups quinoa
1 cup brown rice
3 cups whole-wheat flour
12 ounces whole-wheat penne or other short pasta

Condiments
2 tablespoons apple cider vinegar
3½ tablespoons balsamic vinegar
¼ teaspoon Dijon mustard
¼ cup plus 2 tablespoons low-sodium soy sauce
2 tablespoons white wine vinegar

Beans
1 (15-ounce) can cannellini beans
2 (15-ounce) cans chickpeas
1 (15-ounce) can black beans
1½ cups dried red lentils

Dried Fruit, Nut, and Seed Butters
1 cup sliced almonds
3 cups roasted unsalted almonds
2 cups plus 2 tablespoons unsweetened shredded coconut
½ cup pitted dates
1½ cups all-natural peanut butter
2¾ cups pecans
1 cup raisins
2 tablespoons tahini
⅓ cup walnut pieces

Frozen Produce
1½ pounds frozen corn kernels
10 ounces frozen chopped spinach
1 pound frozen strawberries

Other
1 teaspoon baking soda
1 tablespoon baking powder
7 cups broth (vegetable or chicken)
½ cup plus 3 tablespoons unsweetened cocoa powder
1 (14-ounce) can full-fat coconut milk
3 (28-ounce) cans crushed tomatoes
6 sun-dried tomatoes
1 tablespoon plus 2¼ teaspoons vanilla extract
1 packet quick-rising yeast

Week One Shopping List

Vegetables
2 red bell peppers
3 jalapeño peppers
2 medium cucumbers
1 small head green cabbage
7 medium carrots
1 head cauliflower
4-inch piece fresh ginger
4 butter or Bibb lettuce leaves
1 pound fingerling potatoes
5 cups fresh spinach
6 medium tomatoes
3 cups cherry tomatoes
4 medium zucchini

Herbs
1 bunch fresh basil
1 bunch fresh cilantro
1 bunch fresh flat-leaf parsley

Fruit
1 large apple
5 bananas
2 pints fresh blueberries (or 1 pound frozen)
3 lemons
2 limes

Meat and Fish
1 whole chicken, about 4 pounds
4 pork chops
1½ pounds flank steak
1 pound peeled and deveined shrimp

Dairy
6 ounces whipped cream cheese
26 eggs
8 ounces feta cheese
14 ounces goat cheese
1 pint plain Greek yogurt
6 ounces sour cream

Miscellaneous
3¼ cups plus 2 tablespoons unsweetened almond milk
16 corn tortillas
3 cups salsa verde or tomatillo salsa
2 (12-ounce) packages silken tofu
4 whole-wheat tortillas
2 whole-wheat pita breads
1 loaf of whole-grain bread

Prep Ahead for Week One

- Make the Homemade Cinnamon Granola (page 61) for Day Two.
- Make the marinade for the Sesame-Soy Marinated Flank Steak with Wasabi-Spiked Cauliflower Purée (page 190) and marinate the steak in it for Day Three.
- Make the Spicy Tomato Sauce (page 221) for Days Four and Six.

Week Two

Congratulations! You've made it through Week One. But as Week Two begins, you may be feeling your initial enthusiasm beginning to flag. Take a moment to pat yourself on the back for having come this far, and remind yourself that, from here on out, it will only get easier.

Last week you did a major shopping trip and stocked up on all sorts of new and perhaps unfamiliar pantry items. That was a lot of work, not to mention a financial investment, but this week you're in luck because you've already got many of the pantry items you need. This week's recipes use many of the same ingredients as last week's, so your shopping trip will be much easier to manage.

Like last week, the recipes in this week's meal plan have been designed to use many of the same ingredients to minimize waste and make shopping easier. And again, some recipes are designed specifically to generate leftovers that you can use for another meal later in the week.

Week Two Menu at a Glance

Day One
BREAKFAST Ginger Berry Smoothie

LUNCH Spicy Black Bean Soup with Vegetables

DINNER Tandoori-Spiced Chicken Breast with Crisp Cucumber Salad (enough chicken for two lunches)

DESSERT Yogurt Blueberry Ice Pops

Day Two
BREAKFAST Breakfast Tacos with Green Chiles, Goat Cheese, and Salsa Verde (use leftover Salsa Verde from Week One, Day Two)

LUNCH Roasted Butternut Squash Salad with Goat Cheese, Walnuts, and Balsamic Vinaigrette

DINNER Quinoa-Stuffed Peppers with Black Beans and Yogurt Dressing

DESSERT Berry Crumb Cake (left over from Week One)

Day Three
BREAKFAST Banana Blueberry Whole-Grain Pancakes

LUNCH Curried Chicken Salad Lettuce Wraps with Homemade Mayonnaise

DINNER Garlic-Broiled Shrimp and Peppers over Quinoa (use quinoa left over from Day Two)

DESSERT Peanut Butter Oatmeal Cookies

Day Four
BREAKFAST Scrambled Egg, Goat Cheese, and Cherry Tomato Pita Sandwich

LUNCH Shrimp Salad over Greens with Yogurt Dressing

DINNER Spinach and White Bean Enchiladas with Cashew Cheese

DESSERT Apple Crisp with Fresh Ginger

Day Five

BREAKFAST Whole-Wheat Maple Cinnamon Rolls (leftover from Week One)
LUNCH Brussels Sprouts and Chickpea Salad with Dried Cranberries
DINNER Balsamic-Glazed Wild Salmon with Garlicky Sautéed Spinach
DESSERT Cocoa Almond Pudding

Day Six

BREAKFAST Overnight Cinnamon Oatmeal
LUNCH Garden Salad with Chicken and Balsamic Vinaigrette (use leftover chicken from Day One)
DINNER Grilled Pineapple and Pork Skewers
DESSERT Rich Chocolate Fudge

Day Seven

BREAKFAST Sweet Quinoa Breakfast Cups (use quinoa left over from Day Two)
LUNCH Spiced Chicken Wraps with Yogurt Dressing and Fresh Mint (use leftover chicken from Day One)
DINNER Vegetable Stew
DESSERT Banana Maple Nut "Ice Cream"

SNACKS (CHOOSE ONE OR TWO EACH DAY)

- Celery with goat cheese
- Veggie sticks (carrots, celery, bell peppers) with plain yogurt mixed with curry powder
- Pitted dates stuffed with almonds
- Hard-boiled egg and a small serving of fruit (handful of berries, apricot, tangerine)
- Dried apricots spread with goat cheese
- Smoked salmon on cucumber rounds
- Natural smoked (nitrate-free) turkey or beef jerky
- Leftover chicken or turkey rolled up in lettuce leaves with avocado slices and salsa
- Carrots sticks with hummus
- Oven-Baked Sweet Potato Fries*
- Creamy Peanut Butter–Yogurt Dip* with fresh fruit
- Apple Walnut Bars*

*Recipe included in recipe section

From the Pantry

Oils
1 cup plus 3 tablespoons coconut oil
2¼ cups olive oil

Herbs and Spices
Salt
Black peppercorns
3 onions
16 garlic cloves
1 tablespoon plus ¼ teaspoon cayenne pepper
2 tablespoons chili powder
4 teaspoons ground cinnamon
½ teaspoon ground coriander
4 tablespoons plus 1½ teaspoons ground cumin
4 teaspoons smoked paprika

Sweeteners
2¼ cups coconut sugar
1½ cups honey
½ cup maple syrup

Flours and Grains
2⅓ cup almond flour
3 tablespoons arrowroot starch
½ cup ground flaxseed
1 cup oat flour
6 cups plus 2 tablespoons old-fashioned rolled oats
2½ cups quinoa
3 cups whole-wheat flour

Condiments
1 tablespoon apple cider vinegar
½ cup balsamic vinegar
1 cup Dijon mustard
3 tablespoons low-sodium soy sauce
2 tablespoons white wine vinegar

Dried Fruit, Nut and Seed Butters
½ cup unsweetened shredded coconut
¼ cup dried cranberries
2 cups pitted dates
2¼ cups all-natural peanut butter
½ cup raisins
3⅓ cups walnuts

Beans and Legumes
3 (15-ounce) cans black beans
1 (15-ounce) can cannellini beans

Frozen Produce
3½ cups frozen blueberries
2 cups frozen green beans
1 cup frozen corn
2 (10-ounce) packages chopped frozen spinach
2 cups frozen strawberries

Other
6½ teaspoons baking powder
1 teaspoon baking soda
1 (15-ounce) canned chickpeas
1 cup unsweetened cocoa powder
1 (2-ounce) can diced green chiles

1 (15-ounce) can unsweetened pineapple chunks in their juice
2 (28-ounce) cans tomatillos
1 (14½-ounce) can diced tomatoes
¼ cup tomato paste
1 tablespoon plus 1¼ teaspoons vanilla extract
9½ cups vegetable broth

Week Two Shopping List

Vegetables
1 ripe avocado
20 medium Brussels sprouts
2 small butternut squash
6 carrots
3 cucumbers
¼ cup plus 3 tablespoons grated fresh ginger
3 to 5 jalapeño peppers
1 bunch kale
3 heads butter or Bibb lettuce
5 large red bell peppers
1 pound plus 1 cup fresh spinach
1 pint cherry tomatoes
2 large tomatoes
4 large sweet potatoes

Herbs
2 cups plus 2 tablespoons chopped fresh cilantro
¼ cup chopped fresh mint leaves

Fruit
9 apples (like McIntosh or Fuji)
9 bananas
4 lemons
1 lime

Meat and Fish
3¼ pounds skinless, boneless chicken breast
1½ pounds boneless pork loin, cut into 1½-inch chunks
4 (6-ounce) wild salmon fillets
2¼ pounds peeled and deveined shrimp

Eggs and Dairy
21 eggs
13 ounces goat cheese
1½ cups plus 1 tablespoon milk
8⅓ cups plain yogurt

Miscellaneous
5 cups unsweetened almond milk
½ cup silken tofu
12 corn tortillas
8 slices whole-grain bread
1 whole-wheat pita bread (buy a package of eight and freeze extras for future meals)
4 whole-wheat tortillas

Prep Ahead for Week Two

- Marinate the chicken for Tandoori-Spiced Chicken Breast (page 170) for Day One.

- Prepare Roasted Butternut Squash for Day Two:

    2 small butternut squash, halved lengthwise and seeded
    ¼ teaspoon salt
    ¼ teaspoon freshly ground black pepper

    1. Preheat the oven to 400°F.

    2. Place the squash halves cut-side up on a large baking sheet. Season with the salt and pepper. Roast for 25 minutes, until tender. Let cool.

    3. Cut off the skin and dice the flesh. Store in the refrigerator until ready to use, up to 1 week.

- Make the Yogurt Dressing (page 216) for Days Two and Four.

Week Three

You've made it through a second week of clean eating. It hasn't always been easy, but you are probably starting to feel some of the benefits. Your digestion may have improved, your skin may be clearer, you may have even lost a pound or two (or more). And you're probably starting to get the hang of this clean eating thing.

Again, this week you'll use a lot of the same pantry items as in the previous two weeks. You may be running low on a few frequently used items—like olive oil, garlic, oats, and almonds. Take a few minutes before you do your shopping to take stock of what's in your pantry for this week's recipes.

You may be getting a bit tired of doing so much cooking, but this week you have the benefit of your previous weeks' work. Several meals will be composed partially or entirely from dishes you made in previous weeks and stashed in the pantry, refrigerator, or freezer.

Let yourself glide through the week with the knowledge that you are more than halfway through this four-week meal plan.

Week Three Menu at a Glance

Day One

BREAKFAST No-Bake Coconut Granola Bars

LUNCH Spicy Southwestern Corn and Bean Salad

DINNER Balsamic-Roasted Vegetables with Quinoa

DESSERT Berry Crumb Cake (left over from Week One)

Day Two

BREAKFAST Bacon-Crusted Mini Quiches with Mushrooms and Greens

LUNCH Roasted Vegetable Pitas with Pesto Mayonnaise (leftover roasted vegetables from Day One)

DINNER Pork Fried Brown Rice with Pineapple and Cashews

DESSERT Apple Crisp with Fresh Ginger

Day Three

BREAKFAST Whole-Wheat Blueberry Muffins with Cinnamon-Sugar Topping (left over from Week One)

LUNCH Spicy Black Bean Soup with Vegetables (left over from Week Two)

DINNER Chickpea Tostadas with Cashew Cheese

DESSERT Molten Chocolate Cakes

Day Four

BREAKFAST Overnight Cinnamon Oatmeal

LUNCH Quinoa Salad with Cannellini Beans, Tomatoes, and Lemon Vinaigrette

DINNER Korean Stir-Fried Pork with Brown Rice

DESSERT Yogurt Blueberry Ice Pops

Day Five

BREAKFAST Homemade Cinnamon Granola (left over from Week One)
LUNCH Egg Salad Sandwich with Greek Yogurt and Dill
DINNER Chicken and White Bean Chili
DESSERT Peanut Butter Oatmeal Cookies (left over from Week One)

Day Six

BREAKFAST Bacon-Crusted Mini Quiches with Mushrooms and Greens (left over from Day Two)
LUNCH Caprese Salad with Balsamic Vinaigrette
DINNER Italian Fish Stew
DESSERT Rich Chocolate Fudge (left over from Week Two)

Day Seven

BREAKFAST No-Bake Coconut Granola Bars (left over from Day One)
LUNCH Fresh Herb Frittata with Peas, Bacon, and Feta Cheese
DINNER Thai-Style Curried Chicken Burgers
DESSERT Cocoa Almond Pudding

SNACKS (CHOOSE ONE OR TWO EACH DAY)

- Pitted dates stuffed with almonds
- Hard-boiled egg with salt or spices
- Turkey spread with Homemade Mayonnaise (page 217) and rolled up around cherry tomatoes and basil
- Small apple with nut butter
- Plain yogurt with a drizzle of honey or maple syrup and a handful of chopped nuts
- Celery with peanut butter
- Lightly salted edamame
- Hummus with veggie sticks
- Smoked salmon on cucumber rounds
- Honey Sesame Crackers*
- Pineapple Coconut Trail Mix*
- Smoky-Sweet Chili Almonds*

Recipe included in recipe section

From the Pantry

Oils
¼ cup plus 3 tablespoons coconut oil
1½ cups plus 3 tablespoons plus 2 teaspoons olive oil
1 tablespoon plus 1 teaspoon sesame oil

Herbs and Spices
Salt
Black peppercorns
5 onions
18 garlic cloves
1 tablespoon plus ½ teaspoon cayenne pepper
1½ teaspoons ground cinnamon
4½ teaspoons ground cumin
1 tablespoon chili powder
1 teaspoon dried dill
1 tablespoon dried oregano
2 teaspoons smoked paprika
1 to 2 tablespoons Thai red curry paste

Sweeteners
½ cup plus 2 tablespoons coconut sugar
3½ cups plus 1 tablespoon plus 1 teaspoon honey

Flours and Grains
3 tablespoons arrowroot starch
1 cup brown rice
½ cup ground flaxseed
4¼ cups old-fashioned rolled oats
2½ cups quinoa
½ cup plus 2 tablespoons whole-wheat flour

Condiments
¼ cup plus 3 tablespoons balsamic vinegar
½ cup plus 1 tablespoon plus ¼ teaspoon Dijon mustard
½ cup plus 2 tablespoons low-sodium soy sauce
3 tablespoons plus 1 teaspoon white wine vinegar

Dried Fruit, Nut and Seed Butters
5½ cups chopped almonds
1¼ cups cashews
1¼ cups unsweetened shredded coconut
1 cup dried cranberries
1 cup dried pineapple
1 cup sesame seeds
1⅓ cups chopped walnut pieces

Beans and Legumes
1 (15-ounce) can black beans
2 (15-ounce) cans cannellini beans
1 (15-ounce) can chickpeas

Frozen Produce
1 cup frozen blueberries
1 cup frozen corn kernels
2 cups frozen peas

Other
2 (14-ounce) cans chicken broth
1 (4-ounce) can diced green chiles
¾ cup plus 1 tablespoon unsweetened cocoa powder
¼ cup plus 2 tablespoons nutritional yeast
1 (28-ounce) can diced tomatoes
1 tablespoon plus 1 teaspoon vanilla extract

Week Three Shopping List

Vegetables
2 medium carrots
2 tablespoons plus 1 teaspoon fresh ginger
1 jalapeño pepper
1 head butter or Bibb lettuce
12 ounces button or cremini mushrooms
1 red onion
3½ red or yellow bell peppers
1 pound Swiss chard
14 medium tomatoes
2 small zucchini

Herbs
2½ cups fresh basil
¼ cup plus 2 tablespoons fresh cilantro
2 tablespoons chopped fresh mint

Fruit
4 apples
3 lemons
2 limes

Meat and Fish
12 strips natural smoked bacon
1¼ pounds ground chicken
1 pound boneless skinless chicken breast
2 pounds boneless pork loin
1 pound white fish (cod, halibut) fillets

Eggs and Dairy
32 eggs
10 ounces goat cheese
3 cups plain Greek yogurt
2 tablespoons milk
12 ounces fresh mozzarella

Miscellaneous
3 cups unsweetened almond milk
8 corn tortillas
8 slices whole-grain bread

Prep Ahead for Week Three

- Make the Homemade Mayonnaise (page 217) for Days Two and Five.
- Make the Fresh Basil Pesto (page 219) for Day Two (and also for Week Four, Day Six) and the Pesto White Bean Spread (page 124) for Week Four.
- Make the Cashew Cheese for Day Three (page 224).
- Hard-boil the eggs for Day Five and make a few extra for snacks:

    1. Place 8 (or more) eggs in a large saucepan with cold water to cover. Bring the water to a boil over high heat; then reduce the heat to medium-low and simmer for 13 minutes.

    2. While the eggs are simmering, prepare an ice bath by filling a large bowl halfway with ice cubes and then adding cold water to cover.

    3. Drain the eggs and put them into the ice bath until completely cooled. Refrigerate until ready to use.

Week Four

You're in the home stretch! You've completed three weeks of clean eating and you have one more week to go to complete this four-week meal plan. Over the past three weeks, you've begun to develop not just new eating habits, but new shopping and cooking habits, too. In this final week of the meal plan, these habits will solidify and you'll find that clean eating is beginning to come naturally to you. If you stick with the general clean eating guidelines through this week and beyond, these habits will serve you well for years to come.

You may be wondering how you'll continue your clean eating lifestyle when you no longer have a day-by-day meal plan to guide you. But have confidence that you now have the skills you need to shop clean, cook clean, and eat clean every day.

You may have found some favorite new recipes through the meal plan, which you will want to make again and again. There are also several recipes in the book—particularly in the dinner sections—that were not used in the meal plan, so there's plenty more for you to explore. The Resources section (page 230) lists numerous publications and websites where you can find plenty of clean eating recipes and advice. And Appendix A (page 227) offers tips for eating clean when you dine out.

Week Four Menu at a Glance

Day One

BREAKFAST Protein-Packed Freezer Waffles (or Pancakes) (left over from Week One)

LUNCH Korean Pork Lettuce Wraps with Fresh Herbs (pork left over from Week Three)

DINNER Brussels Sprouts Hash with Caramelized Onions and Poached Eggs

DESSERT Peanut Butter Oatmeal Cookies (left over from Week One)

Day Two

BREAKFAST Red Pepper, Spinach, and Goat Cheese Frittata Bites

LUNCH Fresh Herb Frittata with Peas, Bacon, and Feta Cheese (left over from Week Three)

DINNER Roasted Chicken Breasts with Mustard and Greens

DESSERT Banana Chocolate Tart

Day Three

BREAKFAST Overnight Cinnamon Oatmeal

LUNCH Curried Chicken Salad Lettuce Wraps with Homemade Mayonnaise (prep mayonnaise ahead)

DINNER Oven-Roasted Monkfish and Asparagus with Romesco Sauce

DESSERT Rich Chocolate Fudge (left over from Week Two)

Day Four

BREAKFAST Red Pepper, Spinach, and Goat Cheese Frittata Bites (left over from Day Two)

LUNCH Quinoa Salad with Cannellini Beans, Tomatoes, and Lemon Vinaigrette

DINNER Lamb Loin Chops with Yogurt-Mint Sauce

DESSERT Mini Cheesecakes in Caramel Sauce

Day Five

BREAKFAST Sweet Quinoa Breakfast Cups (left over from Week Two)
LUNCH Smoky Red Lentil Soup with Greens
DINNER Risotto with Mushrooms and Peas
DESSERT Apple Crisp with Fresh Ginger

Day Six

BREAKFAST Homemade Cinnamon Granola (left over from Week One)
LUNCH Egg Salad Sandwich with Greek Yogurt and Dill
DINNER Turkey Meatballs with Whole-Wheat Spaghetti and Spicy Tomato Sauce (pesto [in meatballs] and tomato sauce left over from Week One)
DESSERT Banana Chocolate Tart (left over from Day Two)

Day Seven

BREAKFAST Poached Eggs and Asparagus on Whole-Grain Toast
LUNCH Brussels Sprouts and Chickpea Salad with Dried Cranberries
DINNER Pumpkin and Chickpea Curry
DESSERT Cocoa Almond Pudding

SNACKS (CHOOSE ONE OR TWO EACH DAY)

- Roasted almonds and dried pineapple
- Celery sticks with all-natural nut butter and dried fruit
- Banana with peanut butter
- Hard-boiled egg dipped in Homemade Mayonnaise (page 217) or Romesco Sauce (page 220)
- Basil leaf wraps with goat cheese and cherry tomatoes
- Veggie sticks with Romesco Sauce (page 220)
- Plain Greek yogurt with Homemade Cinnamon Granola (page 61) or fresh fruit
- Walnuts and raisins
- Whole-grain toast with peanut butter and sliced apples
- Tropical Sweet Bars*
- Pesto White Bean Spread*
- Banana Nut Bread*

*Recipe included in recipe section

From the Pantry

Oils
¼ cups plus 3 tablespoons coconut oil
2¼ cups plus 1 tablespoon plus 2 teaspoons olive oil

Herbs and Spices
Salt
Black peppercorns
6 onions
12 garlic cloves
¾ teaspoon cayenne pepper
2¼ teaspoons ground cinnamon
2 teaspoons ground cumin
2 tablespoons curry powder
1 teaspoon dried dill
1 tablespoon plus 1 teaspoon smoked paprika
1 teaspoon ground turmeric

Sweeteners
⅔ cup plus 2 tablespoons coconut sugar
1¾ cups plus 1 tablespoon plus 1 teaspoon honey
½ cup plus 1 tablespoon maple syrup

Flours and Grains
1½ cups almond flour
1 cup Arborio rice
3 tablespoons arrowroot starch
½ cup ground flaxseed
5¼ cups old-fashioned rolled oats
2 cups quinoa
2 cups plus 2 tablespoons whole-wheat flour
8 ounces whole-wheat spaghetti

Condiments
2 tablespoons plus 1 teaspoon apple cider vinegar
Chili paste (optional)
¾ cup plus ¼ teaspoon Dijon mustard
1 tablespoon plus 1 teaspoon white wine vinegar

Dried Fruit, Nut and Seed Butters
1¼ cup chopped almonds
2 cups cashews
1¼ cups dried cranberries
½ cup unsweetened shredded coconut
½ cup pitted dates
½ cup raisins
1 cup chopped walnuts

Beans and Legumes
2 (15-ounce) cans cannellini beans
2 (15-ounce) cans chickpeas
1½ cups red lentils

Frozen Produce
2¾ cups frozen peas

Other
1 tablespoon baking powder
½ teaspoon baking soda
1 cup plus 2 tablespoons unsweetened cocoa powder
3½ teaspoons vanilla extract
2 (14½-ounce) cans diced tomatoes
1 (8-ounce) jar roasted red bell peppers
7½ cups vegetable broth

Week Four Shopping List

Vegetables
2 pounds asparagus
2½ pounds Brussels sprouts
3 carrots
1 small cucumber
2 tablespoons minced fresh ginger
12 large lettuce leaves, such as butter or Bibb
1 pound button or cremini mushrooms
1 pumpkin
6 cups fresh spinach leaves
2 pounds Swiss chard
5 medium tomatoes

Herbs
½ cup fresh basil
1 cup plus 2 tablespoons fresh mint

Fruit
6 large apples (such as McIntosh or Fuji)
1 banana
7 lemons

Meat and Fish
4 bone-in chicken breast halves and 4 bone-in chicken thighs
4 (2-inch-thick) lamb loin chops, or 8 (1-inch-thick) lamb loin chops, about 1½ pounds total
4 (6-ounce) monkfish fillets
¾ pound ground turkey

Eggs and Dairy
12 strips natural smoked bacon
47 eggs
4 ounces feta cheese
24 ounces plain Greek yogurt
6 ounces whipped cream cheese

Miscellaneous
3 cups plus 2 tablespoons unsweetened almond milk
18 ounces silken tofu
12 slices whole-grain bread

Prep Ahead for Week Four

- Make the Homemade Mayonnaise (page 217) for Days Three and Six.
- Make the Lemon Vinaigrette (page 215) for Day Four.
- Prepare the hard-boiled eggs (page 50) for Day Six and make a few extra for snacks.

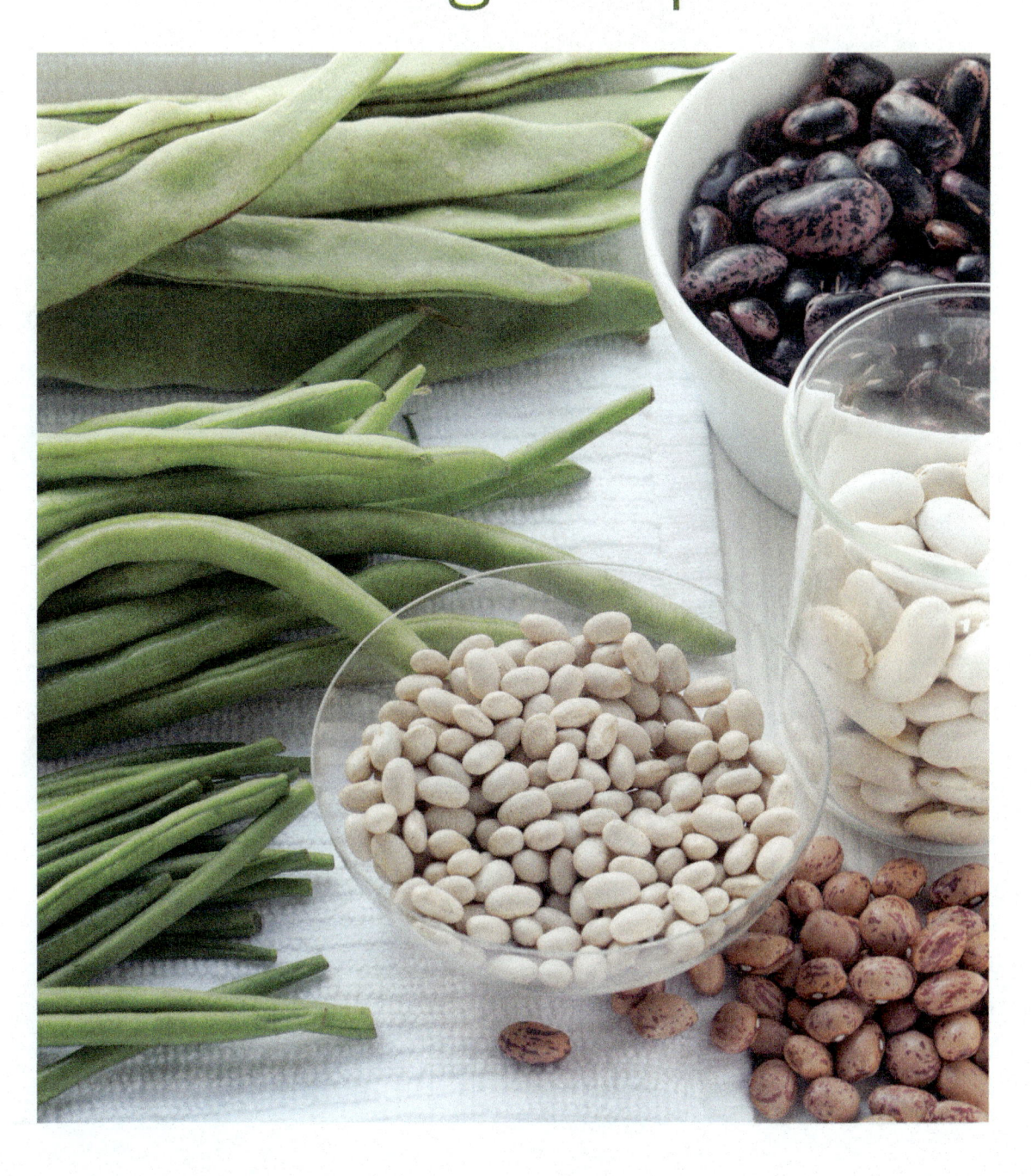

PART TWO
Clean Eating Recipes

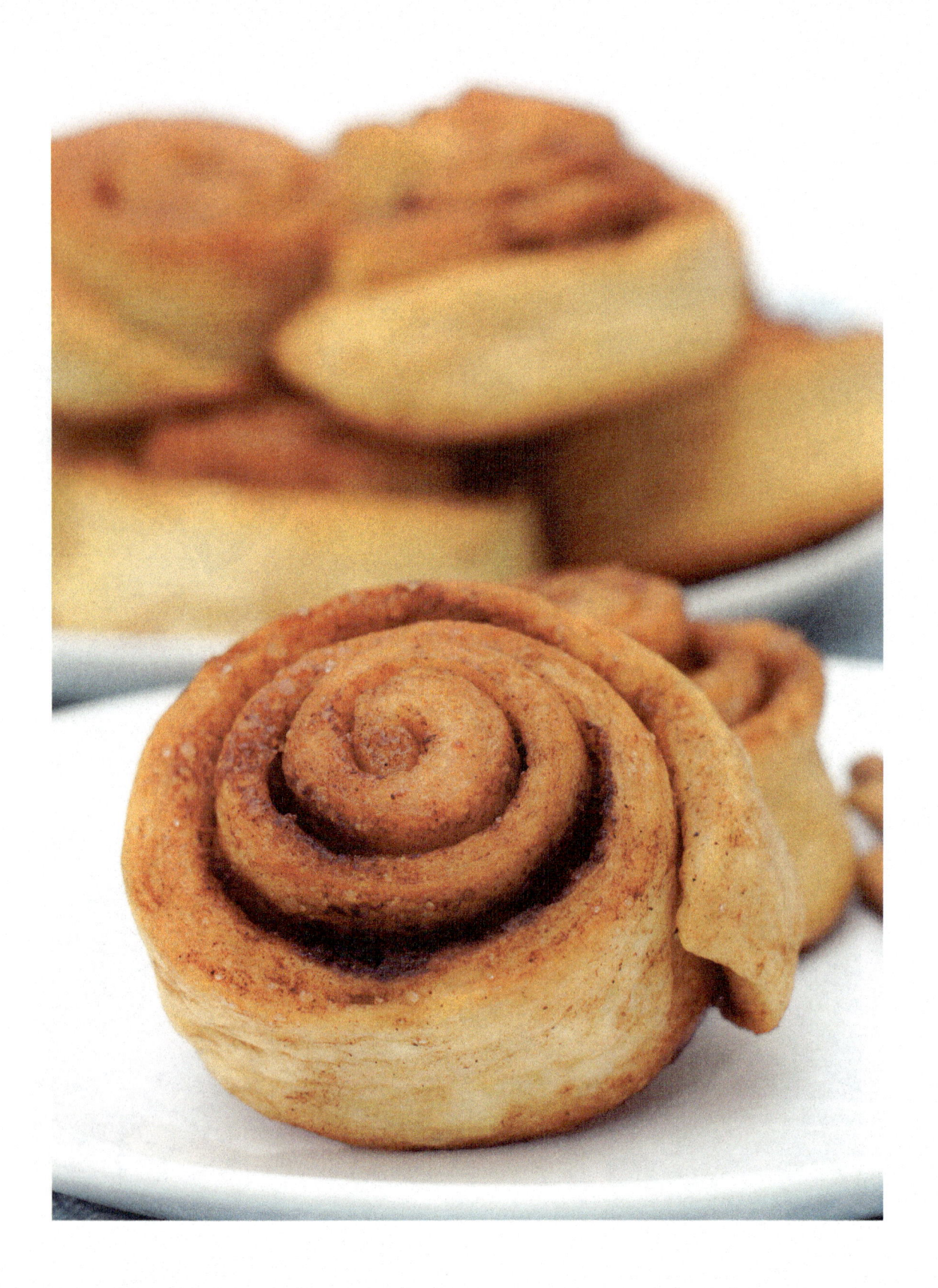

4

Breakfast

Ginger Berry Smoothie   60
Homemade Cinnamon Granola   61
No-Bake Coconut Granola Bars   63
Overnight Cinnamon Oatmeal   65
Protein-Packed Freezer Waffles (or Pancakes)   66
Whole-Wheat Maple Cinnamon Rolls   68
Whole-Wheat Blueberry Muffins with Cinnamon-Sugar Topping   70
Sweet Quinoa Breakfast Cups   72
Banana Blueberry Whole-Grain Pancakes   74
Red Pepper, Spinach, and Goat Cheese Frittata Bites   76
Scrambled Egg, Goat Cheese, and Cherry Tomato Pita Sandwich   77
Breakfast Tacos with Green Chiles, Goat Cheese, and Salsa Verde   79
Poached Eggs in Spicy Tomato Sauce   81
Poached Eggs and Asparagus on Whole-Grain Toast   82
Bacon-Crusted Mini Quiches with Mushrooms and Greens   84

Ginger Berry Smoothie

VEGETARIAN   VEGAN   GLUTEN-FREE   DAIRY-FREE

Prep time: 5 minutes   **Cooking time:** None

A bright kick of ginger in this nutritious smoothie will snap you out of your morning doldrums. Flavored with strawberries and bananas and enriched with almond milk and silken tofu, it's got all the vitamins, protein, and fiber you need. If you prefer, for the almond milk you can substitute another type of nondairy milk—such as coconut, hemp, rice, or soy. Just be sure to check the protein content and add more tofu if needed, since some nondairy milks, like coconut, are not as high in protein.

- 2 cups frozen strawberries
- 1 large banana
- 1½ cups chilled unsweetened almond milk (or other nondairy milk substitute)
- ½ cup silken tofu
- 1½ tablespoons honey
- 2 teaspoons finely grated fresh ginger
- 2 teaspoons fresh lemon juice

In a blender, add the strawberries, banana, almond milk, tofu, honey, ginger, and lemon juice and blend until smooth. If the consistency is too thick, add a bit of water or a splash more of almond milk. Serve immediately.

Serves 2 / Per Serving Calories: 209   Total fat: 2.9g   Saturated fat: 0g   Protein: 3.5g   Carbohydrates: 44.1g   Fiber: 6.1g   Cholesterol: 0mg

> **ON-THE-GO TIP**
>
> Pour the smoothie into a travel cup with a lid so you can sip it on your commute. You can even make the smoothie the night before, pour it into your travel mug, and keep it in the refrigerator until morning. Then briskly shake it before you drink it.

Homemade Cinnamon Granola

VEGETARIAN   VEGAN   GLUTEN-FREE   DAIRY-FREE

Prep time: 15 minutes   **Cook time:** 55 minutes

Often loaded with refined sugar and unhealthful fats, store-bought granola may also include other ingredients not on the clean eating plan. Making your own is easy, and it puts you in control of what goes in it. This recipe is easy to customize, so feel free to substitute different nuts or spices or add dried fruit.

- 5 cups old-fashioned rolled oats
- 1½ cups unsweetened shredded coconut
- 1 cup sliced almonds
- ¼ cup coconut oil, melted
- 5 tablespoons maple syrup
- 2 tablespoons coconut sugar
- 1 tablespoon vanilla extract
- 1½ teaspoons ground cinnamon
- 1 teaspoon salt

1. Preheat the oven to 325°F. Line a large baking sheet with parchment paper.

2. In a large mixing bowl, add the oats, coconut, and almonds and stir together.

3. In a medium bowl, stir together the coconut oil, maple syrup, coconut sugar, vanilla, cinnamon, and salt. Drizzle the coconut oil mixture over the oats mixture and stir to coat evenly. Pour the mixture into the prepared baking sheet and spread out in an even layer. ▶

Homemade Cinnamon Granola, continued

4. Bake for about 45 minutes, until it begins to turn golden brown. Let the granola cool on the baking sheet for at least 1 hour. When cool, break the granola up into small pieces.

Makes about 8 cups (sixteen ½-cup servings) **/ Per Serving** Calories: 253   Total fat: 14.1g   Saturated fat: 8.7g   Protein: 5.4g   Carbohydrates: 26.8g   Fiber: 4.9g   Cholesterol: 0mg

> STORAGE TIP
>
> This recipe makes a large amount of granola. Store the extra in an airtight container at room temperature for up to 2 weeks. You can also freeze the granola in an airtight container or resealable plastic bag for up to 3 months. Bring to room temperature before serving.

No-Bake Coconut Granola Bars

VEGETARIAN   GLUTEN-FREE   DAIRY-FREE

Prep time: 10 minutes (plus overnight to freeze)   **Cooking time:** 3 minutes

Full of protein, these tasty bars take only minutes to make. You can substitute any nut you like. Keep a bag of these in the freezer, and you'll always have a healthful breakfast or snack on hand.

Coconut oil, for the baking dish
1 cup chopped walnuts
1 cup chopped almonds
1 cup dried cranberries
1 cup old-fashioned rolled oats
¾ cup unsweetened shredded coconut
1 teaspoon ground cinnamon
1¼ cups honey
1 teaspoon vanilla extract

1. Lightly coat a 9-by-13-inch baking dish with coconut oil.

2. In a large bowl, stir together the walnuts, almonds, cranberries, oats, coconut, and cinnamon.

3. In a small saucepan, heat the honey and vanilla over medium-high heat for about 3 minutes, stirring frequently, until it boils.

4. Add the hot honey mixture to the walnut mixture and stir to mix well.

5. Quickly transfer the mixture to the prepared baking dish. Cover with a piece of parchment paper and press down on the mixture to pack it tightly into the baking dish. ▸

No-Bake Coconut Granola Bars, continued

6. Transfer the baking dish to the freezer and freeze overnight. Cut into bars and serve chilled. Wrap the leftover bars individually, and store them in the freezer in an airtight container for up to 3 months until ready to serve.

Serves 12 / Per Serving Calories: 266 Fat: 12.2g Saturated fat: 2.2g Protein (grams): 5.4g Carbohydrates (grams): 38.4g Fiber (grams): 3.4g Cholesterol: 17mg

Overnight Cinnamon Oatmeal

VEGETARIAN   GLUTEN-FREE   DAIRY-FREE

Prep time: 5 minutes (plus overnight to soak)   **Cooking time:** None

This super simple recipe—basically oats soaked in almond milk with no cooking whatsoever—is endlessly versatile. You can substitute just about any liquid— coconut milk, soy milk, regular milk, or yogurt, for instance—for the almond milk. And there are many topping possibilities, including fresh fruit, dried fruit, chopped nuts, honey, maple syrup, nut butter, and chia seeds.

- 1 cup old-fashioned rolled oats
- 1 cup unsweetened almond milk
- 2 teaspoons honey
- ½ teaspoon ground cinnamon

In a medium bowl, stir the oats, almond milk, honey, and cinnamon until well combined. Cover with plastic wrap and refrigerate overnight. Bring to room temperature about 15 minutes before serving.

Serves 2 / Per Serving Calories: 193   Total fat: 3.9g   Saturated fat: 0g   Protein: 5.9g   Carbohydrates: 34.4g   Fiber: 4.9g   Cholesterol: 34.4mg

---

ON-THE-GO TIP

Mix the oats in a mason jar for an easy take-along breakfast. You can add toppings either the night before or pop them in just before you leave in the morning.

Protein-Packed Freezer Waffles (or Pancakes)

VEGETARIAN VEGAN DAIRY-FREE

Prep time: 5 minutes   **Cooking time:** 15 minutes

Frozen waffles that can be popped into the toaster make a delicious, healthful, and quick breakfast. These crisp, flavorful vegan waffles are loaded with protein from silken tofu. If you don't have a waffle iron, you can make pancakes instead, using a large nonstick skillet. Reheating pancakes is best done in a toaster oven or oven rather than a pop-up toaster. Top these with a drizzle of honey or maple syrup or fresh fruit.

Coconut oil, for the waffle iron
2 cups whole-wheat flour
1 tablespoon baking powder
1 (12-ounce) package silken tofu
2 tablespoons coconut oil, melted
1 teaspoon apple cider vinegar
1 teaspoon vanilla extract

1. Preheat a waffle iron and brush lightly with coconut oil.

2. In a blender, add the flour, baking powder, tofu, coconut oil, vinegar, and vanilla and blend until smooth.

3. Pour about ¾ cup batter per waffle onto the waffle iron. Close the lid and cook for about 2 minutes, until golden brown. (The waffle will usually quit steaming when it is crisp and ready.)

4. Serve immediately. You can flash freeze the waffles by laying them in a single layer on a baking sheet and placing them in the freezer until frozen. Transfer to resealable plastic bags and store in the freezer for up to 3 months. To serve, pop the frozen waffles into a toaster and heat until hot and crisp.

Makes about 8 waffles or pancakes / Per Serving Calories: 173   Total fat: 4.9g   Saturated fat: 3.2g   Protein: 6.2g   Carbohydrates: 25.8g   Fiber: 0.9g   Cholesterol: 0mg

> ON-THE-GO TIP
>
> To take a waffle with you as you rush out the door, heat it in the toaster, and then wrap it in a napkin to bring along.

Whole-Wheat Maple Cinnamon Rolls

VEGETARIAN   DAIRY-FREE

Prep time: 30 minutes (plus rising time)   **Cooking time:** 30 minutes

These ooey, gooey cinnamon rolls are sure to please the whole family. Made with whole-wheat flour and sweetened with maple syrup, they fit the clean eating plan, but they taste every bit as sinful as those off-limit treats you remember from childhood. Make these ahead of time and heat them up for a few minutes in a hot oven before serving.

1 cup unsweetened almond milk
3 tablespoons coconut oil, plus 5 tablespoons, plus more for the bowl
1 packet quick-rising yeast
¼ cup maple syrup, plus 1 tablespoon
¼ teaspoon salt
3 cups whole-wheat pastry flour, plus more for dusting
1½ teaspoons ground cinnamon

1. In a small saucepan, add the almond milk and 3 tablespoons of the coconut oil and heat over medium heat until the mixture is warm (between 110°F and 115°F on a candy thermometer) and the coconut oil is melted. Pour into a large mixing bowl. If the mixture is hot to the touch, let it cool to warm.

2. Sprinkle the yeast and 1 tablespoon of the maple syrup over the top of the almond-milk mixture and stir gently to combine. Set aside for about 10 minutes, until foamy. Stir in the salt.

3. Add the flour about ½ cup at a time, and stir to combine after each addition. Transfer the dough to a floured surface and knead for about 2 minutes until it forms a smooth ball.

4. Clean the mixing bowl and coat it lightly with coconut oil. Add the dough ball and turn to coat. Cover the bowl with a clean dishtowel and set aside to rise until doubled, about 1 hour.

5. In a small saucepan, melt the remaining 5 tablespoons coconut oil over medium heat. Use about 2 tablespoons of the oil to coat the bottom and sides of an 8-inch square baking pan.

6. Turn the dough out onto a lightly floured work surface and roll out into a rectangle about 14 by 8 inches. Brush the top with 3 tablespoons of the melted coconut oil. Drizzle with the remaining ¼ cup of the maple syrup and sprinkle with the cinnamon.

7. Starting with one of the long sides, roll up the rectangle into a cylinder. With the seam-side down, cut the cylinder with a serrated knife into 1½- to 2-inch rounds. Preheat the oven to 350°F. Place the rounds next to each other in the prepared baking pan, cover, and let rise until doubled, about 30 minutes.

8. Bake the rolls for 25 to 30 minutes, until they turn golden brown. Remove from the oven and let cool for 5 minutes. Serve immediately. Let any extra rolls come to room temperature; then store in an airtight container at room temperature for up to 1 week or freeze for up to 3 months.

Makes 10 rolls / Per Serving Calories: 262 Total fat: 11.6g Saturated fat: 9.5g Protein: 4.2g Carbohydrates: 36g Fiber: 1.4g Cholesterol: 0mg

COOKING TIP

To speed the dough's rise in step 4, set the bowl in a warm place like a sunny spot on your kitchen counter, on top of a warm oven, or on top of your running clothes dryer.

Whole-Wheat Blueberry Muffins with Cinnamon-Sugar Topping

VEGETARIAN

Prep time: 15 minutes   **Cooking time:** 20 minutes

Studded with sweet blueberries and topped with a dusting of cinnamon sugar, these big, fluffy muffins are just the kind of breakfast that will make you excited to get out of bed. They're easy to prepare and a batch will last at least a few days (well, if you're lucky). Make them ahead of time for a healthful grab-and-go breakfast.

Coconut oil, for the pan
¼ cup coconut sugar
¼ teaspoon ground cinnamon
¾ cup unsweetened almond milk
¼ cup cooking oil
¼ cup honey
1 egg, lightly beaten
2 cups whole-wheat flour
1 tablespoon baking powder
½ teaspoon salt
1 cup fresh or frozen organic blueberries (if using frozen, do not thaw)

1. Preheat the oven to 400°F. Lightly coat a 12-cup muffin pan with coconut oil.

2. In a small bowl, stir together the coconut sugar and cinnamon.

3. In a large bowl, add the almond milk, cooking oil, honey, and egg and stir to mix well. Add the flour, baking powder, and salt, and stir just until mixed (the batter should be lumpy). Gently fold in the blueberries.

4. Spoon the batter into the prepared muffin cups, filling about three-quarters full. Sprinkle the cinnamon-sugar mixture over the tops.

5. Bake for about 20 minutes, until the tops are golden brown. Turn out the muffins onto a wire rack to cool. Serve immediately. Store in an airtight container at room temperature for up to 1 week or in the freezer for up to 3 months.

Makes 12 muffins / Per Serving Calories: 174 Total fat: 5.5g Saturated fat: 0.8g Protein: 3.2g Carbohydrates: 28.9g Fiber: 0.9g Cholesterol: 15mg

Sweet Quinoa Breakfast Cups

VEGETARIAN   GLUTEN-FREE   DAIRY-FREE

Prep time: 10 minutes   **Cooking time:** 40 minutes

Crunchy, sweet, and fruity, these tasty bites make a great on-the-go breakfast or snack for busy days. Be sure to make an extra batch to freeze. You can vary the recipe to your liking by substituting different fresh fruits (pears, blueberries, bananas—whatever strikes your fancy) or adding nuts, seeds, or dried fruits.

- 2 cups uncooked quinoa
- Coconut oil, for the pan
- 2 eggs, lightly beaten
- 1 cup chopped apple, such as McIntosh or Fuji
- ½ cup raisins
- 5 tablespoons maple syrup
- 1 cup old-fashioned rolled oats
- ½ teaspoon ground cinnamon

1. In a medium saucepan, add 4 cups of water, stir in the quinoa, and bring to a boil over medium-high heat. Reduce heat to low, cover, and cook for 15 to 20 minutes, until the quinoa is tender. Set aside off the heat, covered, for 5 minutes. Transfer 3 cups of the cooked quinoa to an airtight storage container and store in the refrigerator for other meals that week.

2. Preheat the oven to 350°F. Lightly coat the cups of a 24-cup mini muffin pan with coconut oil.

3. In a large mixing bowl, stir together the eggs, apple, raisins, and maple syrup. Add the 1 cup remaining cooked quinoa, the oats, and cinnamon and stir to combine.

4. Spoon about 1 tablespoon of the mixture into each muffin cup. Bake for 15 to 20 minutes, until golden brown and crisp. Serve warm. To store extras, cool to room temperature and keep in an airtight container in the refrigerator for up to 1 week. Bring to room temperature or warm in the oven before serving. The cups can also be frozen wrapped tightly in plastic wrap for up to 3 months. Defrost overnight in the refrigerator; then bring to room temperature or warm in the oven before serving.

Makes 24 mini cups / Per Serving Calories: 195   Total fat: 3g   Saturated fat: 0.6g   Protein: 5.8g   Carbohydrates: 37.4g   Fiber 3.2g   Cholesterol: 41mg

Banana Blueberry Whole-Grain Pancakes

VEGETARIAN

Prep time: 10 minutes **Cooking time:** 10 minutes

These wholesome pancakes get a nutty flavor from two whole grains—oats and wheat. Sweetened with a touch of honey, mashed banana, and blueberries, they don't even need maple syrup, but feel free to drizzle some on if you like. For a more substantial topping, stir more fresh blueberries into plain yogurt and dollop the mixture on top.

- 1 cup oat flour
- 1 cup whole-wheat flour
- 2¼ teaspoons baking powder
- ½ teaspoon baking soda
- ¼ teaspoon salt
- 2 eggs, lightly beaten
- ¼ cup cooking oil, plus 2 teaspoons
- 1 banana, mashed
- 2 tablespoons honey
- 1½ cups milk
- ½ cup fresh or frozen blueberries (if using frozen, do not thaw)

1. In a large mixing bowl, add the oat flour, whole-wheat flour, baking powder, baking soda, and salt and stir to combine.

2. In a medium bowl, add the eggs, ¼ cup of the cooking oil, banana, honey, and milk and stir to combine. Add the egg mixture to the flour mixture and stir to combine. Gently fold in the blueberries.

3. In a large nonstick skillet, heat the remaining 2 teaspoons of cooking oil over medium-high heat. Pour in ¼ cup of batter for each pancake, leaving room between the pancakes so they are not crowded, and cook until the underside is

golden brown and bubbles appear on the top, about 2 minutes. Flip over and cook until the second side is golden brown, about 2 minutes more. Serve hot. To store leftovers, lay out on a cookie sheet and put in the freezer for 2 hours. Pack into a resealable plastic bag and push the air out. To serve, reheat in the toaster.

....

Serves 6 / Per Serving Calories: 315   Total fat: 13g   Saturated fat: 2.9g   Protein: 8.3g   Carbohydrates: 42.4g   Fiber: 3g   Cholesterol: 60mg

INGREDIENT TIP

You can make your own oat flour out of old-fashioned rolled oats. To make 1 cup of oat flour, in a blender, process 1 cup of rolled oats until it reaches a flourlike consistency.

Red Pepper, Spinach, and Goat Cheese Frittata Bites

VEGETARIAN GLUTEN-FREE

Prep time: 10 minutes   **Cooking time:** 10 minutes

Eggs are a nutritious protein-filled breakfast food, and these bites, filled with veggies and goat cheese, are a delicious rendition. They're scrumptious for a Sunday brunch, and since they are so good at room temperature, they're a convenient quick grab-and-go breakfast.

Coconut oil, for the pan
8 eggs
¼ cup unsweetened almond milk
½ teaspoon salt
½ teaspoon freshly ground black pepper
3 cups gently packed chopped fresh spinach leaves
1 small red bell pepper, seeded, deribbed, and diced
4 ounces goat cheese, crumbled

1. Preheat the oven to 375°F. Coat a 24-cup mini muffin pan with coconut oil.

2. In a large bowl, whisk together the eggs, almond milk, salt, and pepper. Stir in the spinach, bell pepper, and cheese.

3. Spoon the egg mixture into the prepared muffin cups, filling each almost to the top.

4. Bake for 8 to 10 minutes, until puffed and set in the center. Serve hot. Store extra bites in an airtight container in the refrigerator for up to 5 days or freeze them individually, wrapped tightly in plastic wrap, for up to 3 months. Bring to room temperature before serving.

Makes 24 bites (about 8 servings) / Per Serving Calories: 140   Total fat: 9.8g   Saturated fat: 5.1g   Protein: 10.8g   Carbohydrates: 2.5g   Fiber: 0g   Cholesterol: 180mg

Scrambled Egg, Goat Cheese, and Cherry Tomato Pita Sandwich

VEGETARIAN

Prep time: 5 minutes **Cooking time:** 6 minutes

Scrambled eggs make an ideal weekday breakfast because they're quick to make, loaded with protein, and, of course, delicious and satisfying. This fresh and flavorful scramble takes only minutes to make. Because the eggs are tucked into a pita pocket, the sandwich is easy to take along on your morning commute. Get creative with variations: Add roasted red peppers, chopped chiles, or fresh herbs; switch the goat cheese for feta or ricotta; or top your sandwich with a dollop of salsa.

- 2 whole-wheat pita breads, cut in half
- 4 eggs
- 4 egg whites
- 2 tablespoons unsweetened almond milk
- 6 cherry tomatoes, halved lengthwise
- 1 teaspoon salt
- ½ teaspoon freshly ground black pepper
- 1 tablespoon olive oil
- ½ cup (2 ounces) crumbled goat cheese

1. Preheat the oven to 350°F.

2. Wrap the pita bread in aluminum foil and place in the oven to warm while you cook the eggs.

3. In a medium bowl, whisk together the eggs and egg whites until well combined. Stir in the almond milk, tomatoes, salt, and pepper until combined. ▶

Scrambled Egg, Goat Cheese, and Cherry Tomato Pita Sandwich, continued

4. In a large skillet, heat the olive oil over medium-high heat. Reduce the heat to medium, add the egg mixture, and cook, stirring frequently, until the eggs are set, about 5 minutes. Add the goat cheese and continue to cook, stirring, until the cheese melts, about 1 minute more.

5. Stuff one-fourth of the eggs into each pita bread half and serve immediately.

Serves 4 / Per Serving Calories: 319 Total fat: 17.2g Saturated fat: 7.3g Protein: 18.4g Carbohydrates: 26.2g Fiber: 4.9g Cholesterol: 179mg

ON-THE-GO TIP

If you want to take your pita sandwich with you on your commute, wrap it tightly in aluminum foil. It will keep warm until you're ready to eat. Be sure to bring along a napkin if you plan to eat it on the train or in the car.

Breakfast Tacos with Green Chiles, Goat Cheese, and Salsa Verde

VEGETARIAN   GLUTEN-FREE

Prep time: 10 minutes   **Cooking time:** 10 minutes

A quick scramble, studded with diced green chiles, enriched with creamy goat cheese, and wrapped up in a warm corn tortilla, makes a delicious and satisfying breakfast. Feel free to add more vegetables if you like, such as kale, chard, spinach, diced bell peppers, or scallions. Add them along with the onions. You may have extra Salsa Verde left over from another recipe, but if not, it can be made ahead and kept in the refrigerator until you're ready to use it.

4 corn tortillas
4 eggs, lightly beaten
½ teaspoon salt
¼ teaspoon freshly ground black pepper
2 teaspoons olive oil
¼ cup chopped onion
1 (2-ounce) can diced green chiles
½ cup (2 ounces) goat cheese
½ cup Salsa Verde (page 218)

1. Preheat the oven to 350°F. Wrap the tortillas in aluminum foil and put them in the oven to warm while you prepare the eggs.

2. In a medium bowl, whisk together the eggs, salt, and pepper.

3. In a large skillet, heat the oil over medium-high heat. Add the onions and cook, stirring, until soft, about 5 minutes. Reduce the heat to medium, add the chiles and the egg mixture, and cook, stirring frequently with a silicone spatula, until the eggs are set, about 3 minutes. Stir in the goat cheese and remove from the heat. ▶

Breakfast Tacos with Green Chiles, Goat Cheese, and Salsa Verde, continued

4. Divide the egg mixture evenly among the warm tortillas. Top each with about 2 tablespoons of Salsa Verde. Serve immediately.

Serves 4 / Per Serving Calories: 256   Total fat: 13.3g   Saturated fat: 5.4g   Protein: 13.2g   Carbohydrates: 23.3g   Fiber: 5.9g   Cholesterol: 179mg

> TIP TO DOUBLE THE RECIPE
>
> This recipe serves four, but it is easily halved or doubled. Simply halve or double the ingredients and proceed with the recipe. You may need to use a smaller or larger skillet.

Poached Eggs in Spicy Tomato Sauce

VEGETARIAN   GLUTEN-FREE

Prep time: 5 minutes   **Cooking time:** 8 minutes

Gently poaching eggs in tomato sauce makes a healthful and substantial breakfast, perfect for a chilly morning. Since the recipe uses a make-ahead tomato sauce, it can be put together in just a few minutes. Add a slice of whole-grain toast to sop up the yummy sauce.

- 4 cups Spicy Tomato Sauce (page 221)
- 4 eggs
- 4 slices whole-grain bread
- ½ teaspoon salt
- ½ teaspoon freshly ground black pepper
- 2 tablespoons minced fresh basil

1. In a medium skillet, bring the tomato sauce to a bubbly simmer over medium-high heat.

2. Make four wells in the sauce with the back of a large spoon and crack an egg gently into each of the wells. Reduce the heat to medium-low, and cover and cook for about 6 minutes, until the whites of the eggs are set but the yolks are still runny.

3. Meanwhile, toast the bread.

4. Place one slice of toast on each of four serving plates. Gently scoop an egg, along with some of the sauce, and place it on top of a toast slice. Spoon a bit more sauce over and around the egg. Repeat with the remaining eggs and toast slices. Sprinkle the poached eggs with the salt and pepper, and the basil. Serve immediately.

Serves 4 / Per Serving Calories: 221   Total fat: 6.9g   Saturated fat: 1.6g   Protein: 13.6g   Carbohydrates: 28.8g   Fiber: 7.8g   Cholesterol: 186mg

Poached Eggs and Asparagus on Whole-Grain Toast

VEGETARIAN   DAIRY-FREE

Prep time: 5 minutes   **Cooking time:** 15 minutes

Fresh spring asparagus makes any meal seem like a special occasion. Celebrate the morning with this simple but satisfying breakfast. The still-runny yolks of the poached eggs drizzle over the rest of the dish, making their own sauce and eliminating any need for rich toppings like hollandaise. If asparagus isn't in season, substitute red bell peppers cut into strips or zucchini cut into sticks and adjust the cooking time as needed. Make sure the bread you choose is made of 100 percent whole grains.

- 4 slices whole-grain bread
- 1 pound asparagus, trimmed
- 2 tablespoons olive oil
- ½ teaspoon salt, plus more for serving
- ½ teaspoon freshly ground black pepper, plus more for serving
- 8 eggs

1. Preheat the broiler. Set a large skillet half full of water over medium-high heat and bring to a simmer. Reduce the heat to medium-low.

2. Meanwhile, arrange the bread and asparagus on a large baking sheet, drizzle with the olive oil, and sprinkle with the salt and pepper. Broil in the preheated oven for about 1 to 2 minutes, watching carefully so it doesn't burn, until the bread is toasted on top. Flip the bread over and broil another 1 to 2 minutes, until the second side is toasted. Transfer the bread to four serving plates and return the asparagus to the broiler. Broil for an additional 5 to 8 minutes, watching carefully, until tender.

3. Carefully crack the eggs into the skillet of simmering water. Cook for 4 minutes, until the whites are set and the yolks are still runny.

4. Arrange the asparagus on top of the toast slices, dividing equally. Top each with two eggs and a sprinkling of salt and pepper, and serve immediately.

Serves 4 / Per Serving Calories: 299   Fat: 16.4g   Saturated fat: 3.8g   Protein: 17.6g   Carbohydrates: 21.2g   Fiber: 7.4g   Cholesterol: 327mg

COOKING TIP

The key to perfectly poached eggs is to drop the raw eggs into simmering, not boiling water, and then immediately reduce the heat to medium-low to keep the water at a steady simmer (do not let the water boil once the eggs have been added). And crack the eggs into the water starting at 12 o'clock and move counterclockwise. Set a timer for 4 minutes and, using a slotted spoon, remove the eggs promptly, starting with the one at 12 o'clock and moving clockwise.

Bacon-Crusted Mini Quiches with Mushrooms and Greens

GLUTEN-FREE   DAIRY-FREE

Prep time: 10 minutes   **Cooking time:** 40 minutes

These individual quiches replace the usual pastry crust with crisp bacon, making a perfect on-the-go breakfast. Filled with mushrooms and greens, they are hearty and satisfying. If you're feeling decadent, add a few ounces of grated cheese such as Gruyère or fontina, stirring half into the egg mixture and sprinkling the other half over the top to brown.

8 strips natural smoked bacon
1 tablespoon olive oil
1 small onion, chopped
¾ cup chopped button or cremini mushrooms
1 pound Swiss chard, stemmed and cut into ribbons
8 eggs
¾ teaspoon salt
¼ teaspoon freshly ground black pepper

1. Preheat the oven to 350°F. Place a strip of bacon into each of eight cups in a muffin pan, wrapping the bacon around the edge to form a bottomless cup.

2. In a medium skillet, heat the olive oil over medium-high heat. Add the onion and mushrooms and cook, stirring frequently, until they soften, about 3 minutes. Add the chard and cook, tossing frequently, for 3 to 4 minutes more, until wilted.

3. In a large bowl, whisk the eggs with the salt and pepper until frothy. Stir in the vegetable mixture; then ladle the egg-vegetable mixture into the bacon-lined muffin cups, dividing equally.

4. Bake about 30 minutes, until puffed and golden. Serve immediately, or cool to room temperature and store in an airtight container in the refrigerator for up to 5 days or in the freezer for up to 3 months.

Serves 8 / Per Serving Calories: 197   Fat: 14.2g   Saturated fat: 4.2g   Protein: 13.8g   Carbohydrates: 3.9g   Fiber: 1.2g   Cholesterol: 185mg

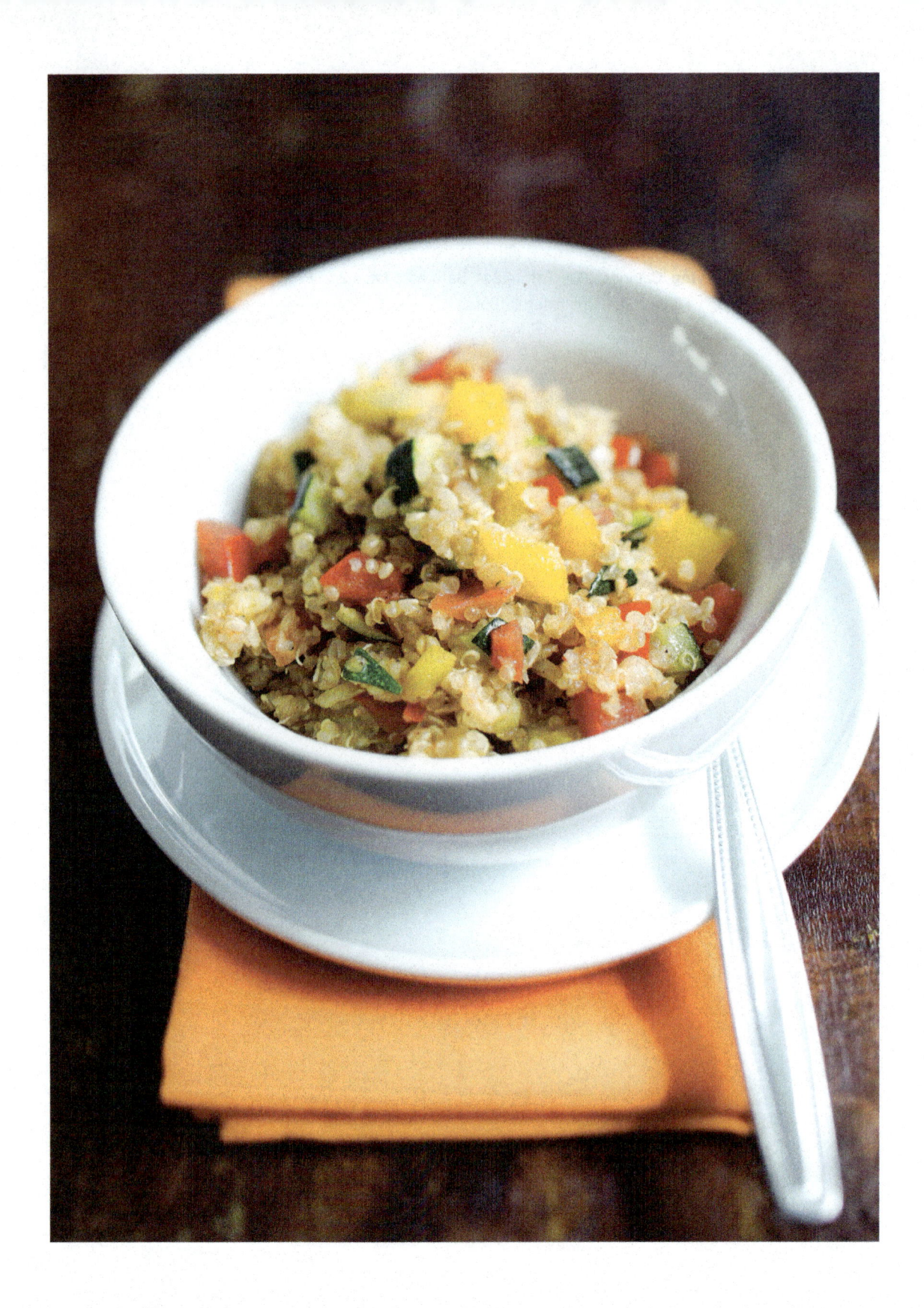

5

Lunch

Fresh Herb Frittata with Peas, Bacon, and Feta Cheese   88
Caprese Salad with Balsamic Vinaigrette   90
Spicy Southwestern Corn and Bean Salad   91
Roasted Butternut Squash Salad with Goat Cheese, Walnuts, and Balsamic Vinaigrette   92
Mediterranean Chickpea Salad with Red Bell Peppers and Feta Cheese   94
Brussels Sprouts and Chickpea Salad with Dried Cranberries   95
Quinoa Salad with Cannellini Beans, Tomatoes, and Lemon Vinaigrette   96
Brown Rice and Black Bean Salad with Spinach and Lemon Vinaigrette   97
Shrimp Salad over Greens with Yogurt Dressing   98
Spinach Salad with Chicken and Sun-Dried Tomato and Basil Vinaigrette   99
Garden Salad with Chicken and Balsamic Vinaigrette   100
Roasted Vegetable Pitas with Pesto Mayonnaise   101
Egg Salad Sandwich with Greek Yogurt and Dill   102
Curried Chicken Salad Lettuce Wraps with Homemade Mayonnaise   103
Spiced Chicken Wraps with Yogurt Dressing and Fresh Mint   104
Korean Pork Lettuce Wraps with Fresh Herbs   105
Smoky Red Lentil Soup with Greens   106
Spicy Black Bean Soup with Vegetables   108

Fresh Herb Frittata with Peas, Bacon, and Feta Cheese

GLUTEN-FREE

Prep time: 5 minutes   **Cooking time:** 20 minutes

Quick to make and endlessly versatile, a frittata is delicious hot, warm, or at room temperature, so it makes a perfect take-along lunch. This version combines fresh mint with bright green peas, salty bacon, and tangy goat cheese. If you can find fresh peas, by all means use them, but frozen peas are perfectly acceptable here.

1 tablespoon olive oil
½ small onion, diced
1 garlic clove, minced
4 strips natural smoked bacon, diced
2 cups frozen peas, thawed
10 eggs
2 tablespoons unsweetened almond milk
¾ teaspoon salt
½ cup (2 ounces) crumbled feta cheese, plus ½ cup
2 tablespoons chopped fresh mint

1. Preheat the oven to 450°F.

2. In a large oven-safe skillet over medium-high heat, heat the olive oil. Add the onion, garlic, and bacon and cook, stirring frequently, for about 5 minutes, until the onion is soft and the bacon is crisp. Stir in the peas and cook 2 minutes more.

3. In a medium bowl, whisk the eggs with the almond milk and salt. Add 2 ounces of the feta cheese and the mint, and whisk to combine. Pour the egg mixture over the vegetables in the skillet.

4. Put the skillet in the oven and cook for 8 to 10 minutes, until the top is nearly set. Crumble the remaining 2 ounces of feta cheese over the top. Set the broiler to high and put the skillet under it. Broil until the cheese turns golden brown,

about 3 minutes. Serve immediately or let cool to room temperature. To store leftovers, cut the frittata into wedges and wrap them in plastic wrap. Refrigerate for up to 5 days or freeze for up to 3 months. Bring to room temperature before serving.

Serves 8 / Per Serving Calories: 238 Fat: 15.8g Saturated Fat: 6.8 Carbohydrates: 7g Protein: 17g Fiber: 2.3g Cholesterol: 230mg

DIET VARIATION

For a vegetarian version, substitute vegetarian bacon or sausage for the regular bacon in this recipe.

Caprese Salad with Balsamic Vinaigrette

VEGETARIAN   GLUTEN-FREE

Prep time: 5 minutes   **Cooking time:** None

This simple salad tastes like summer on a plate. Red, ripe, succulent summer tomatoes are layered with creamy and mild fresh mozzarella and flavorful fresh basil, and then drizzled with simple, sweet-and-savory Balsamic Vinaigrette. Look for the juiciest, ripest (but not overripe) tomatoes you can find for this dish. A whole-grain roll is a great accompaniment since you can use it to soak up all the tasty juices.

- 4 medium tomatoes, sliced into thick rounds
- 12 ounces fresh mozzarella, cut into ¼-inch rounds
- ½ cup fresh basil leaves
- ½ cup Balsamic Vinaigrette (page 214)
- ½ teaspoon salt
- ¼ teaspoon freshly ground black pepper

Arrange the tomato and mozzarella slices in alternating layers on a plate (or in a storage container if you plan to take your lunch to-go). Tuck the basil leaves between the tomato and cheese slices. Drizzle the vinaigrette over the top. Sprinkle with salt and pepper and serve immediately, or refrigerate up to 3 hours until ready to serve.

Serves 4 / Per Serving Calories: 386   Total fat: 15.5g   Saturated fat: 9.1g   Protein: 25.5g   Carbohydrates: 7.9g   Fiber: 1.6g   Cholesterol: 46mg

INGREDIENT TIP

If you can find fresh mozzarella in small balls, called *bocconcini*, use those in place of the sliced cheese and substitute a pint of halved cherry tomatoes for the large tomatoes.

Spicy Southwestern Corn and Bean Salad

VEGETARIAN   VEGAN   GLUTEN-FREE   DAIRY-FREE

Prep time: 10 minutes   **Cooking time:** None

Full of crunchy, flavorful vegetables and loaded with protein from the black beans, this zesty salad makes a perfect lunch by itself, or you can use it as a dip for (clean) tortilla chips. If you can find frozen roasted corn with no additives, it will add a bit of smoky flavor. Or roast the corn kernels yourself by tossing them in a hot skillet with a little cooking oil and a sprinkle of salt, and stirring frequently for about 5 minutes until the corn begins to brown.

- 3 tablespoons freshly squeezed lime juice
- 1 tablespoon olive oil
- ½ teaspoon chili powder
- ½ teaspoon ground cumin
- 1 teaspoon salt
- 1 cup frozen corn kernels (thawed)
- 1 (15-ounce) can black beans, rinsed and drained
- 1½ cups diced fresh tomatoes (3 medium tomatoes)
- ½ small red onion, diced
- 1 jalapeño pepper, seeded and diced
- ¼ cup chopped fresh cilantro

1. To make the dressing, in a small bowl, whisk together the lime juice, olive oil, chili powder, cumin, and salt.

2. In a large bowl, stir together the corn, beans, tomatoes, onion, and jalapeño. Add the dressing and toss to mix well. Sprinkle the cilantro over the top. Serve immediately, or store in the refrigerator in an airtight container for up to 3 days.

Serves 6 / Per Serving Calories: 301   Total fat: 3.7g   Saturated fat: 0.6g   Protein: 16.6g   Carbohydrates: 53.7g   Fiber: 12.3g   Cholesterol: 0mg

Roasted Butternut Squash Salad with Goat Cheese, Walnuts, and Balsamic Vinaigrette

VEGETARIAN   GLUTEN-FREE

Prep time: 10 minutes (plus 20 minutes preparing the squash ahead)   **Cooking time:** None

Roasted butternut squash has a rich, complex sweetness that pairs well with peppery arugula and tangy goat cheese. A simple balsamic vinaigrette and a sprinkling of crunchy walnuts finishes it off. If you're feeling ambitious, you could add a bit of grilled fish or chicken to this salad to make it a heartier meal, but it's really quite perfect as it is.

- 1 head butter or Bibb lettuce (reserve 4 large leaves for Chicken Salad Wraps on Day Three)
- 3 cups roasted butternut squash (prep ahead, page 44)
- ½ cup Balsamic Vinaigrette (page 214)
- ½ cup chopped walnuts
- ½ cup (2 ounces) crumbled goat cheese

In a large bowl, toss the Roasted Butternut Squash and lettuce. Add the Balsamic Vinaigrette and toss to coat. Divide the salad into four individual servings. Garnish with the walnuts and goat cheese, dividing among the salads. Store the salad and dressing separately in the refrigerator in airtight containers up to 3 days.

Serves 4 / Per Serving Calories: 329   Total fat: 26.2g   Saturated fat: 6.1g   Protein: 8g   Carbohydrates: 20.6g   Fiber 4.4g   Cholesterol: 15mg

ON-THE-GO TIP

This salad makes a great take-along lunch, but if you dress it ahead of time, the lettuce will wilt. Instead, pack the salad into pint-size mason jars. First, divide the dressing among the four jars. Next, add the squash, then the lettuce, and finally the nuts and cheese. Cap the jars and you're good to go. When you're ready to eat, pour the contents of the jar out into a serving bowl, toss, and enjoy.

Mediterranean Chickpea Salad with Red Bell Peppers and Feta Cheese

VEGETARIAN   GLUTEN-FREE

Prep time: 10 minutes   **Cooking time:** None

This refreshing and nutritious salad takes just minutes to make. It travels well, too, and even gets better with time, so it's a great take-along lunch. The fresh parsley and lemon give it a distinctive Mediterranean flavor. For variation, you could add halved cherry tomatoes, pitted Kalamata olives, or minced fresh oregano. For a more substantial meal, you might even top the salad with grilled shrimp or fish.

1 (15-ounce) can chickpeas, rinsed and drained
1 red bell pepper, seeded, deribbed, and diced
1 medium cucumber, diced
½ medium red onion, finely chopped
3 tablespoons olive oil
Juice of 1 freshly squeezed lemon
⅓ cup chopped fresh parsley
½ teaspoon salt
¼ teaspoon freshly ground black pepper
1 cup crumbled feta cheese

1. In a large bowl, combine the chickpeas, bell pepper, cucumber, and red onion and toss to mix.

2. Add the olive oil, lemon juice, parsley, salt, and pepper, and toss to combine well.

3. Sprinkle the feta cheese over the top and serve immediately, or cover and refrigerate for up to 2 days.

Serves 6 / Per Serving Calories: 402   Total fat: 16.8g   Saturated fat: 5.2g   Protein: 17.8g   Carbohydrates: 47.9g   Fiber: 13.3g   Cholesterol: 22mg

Brussels Sprouts and Chickpea Salad with Dried Cranberries

VEGETARIAN   GLUTEN-FREE   DAIRY-FREE

Prep time: 10 minutes   **Cooking time:** 8 minutes

Brussels sprouts often get short shrift, but that's probably because they're often cooked until they turn to mush. Slicing them thinly is key to the balance of textures in this salad. Here they are quickly sautéed just until they are tender but still a vibrant green. Their pleasingly bitter flavor pairs well with a slightly citrus-based dressing and sweet, chewy dried cranberries.

- 1 tablespoon coconut oil
- ¼ cup thinly sliced onion
- 4 cups (about 20 medium) very thinly sliced Brussels sprouts
- 1 cup canned chickpeas, rinsed and drained
- ¼ cup dried cranberries
- ½ cup Lemon Vinaigrette (page 215)

1. In a small skillet over medium-high heat, heat the coconut oil. Add the onion and cook, stirring, until the onion is softened, about 5 minutes. Transfer the onion to a small bowl.

2. In the same skillet, add the Brussels sprouts. Cook, stirring, for about 2 minutes, until the sprouts turn bright green and become fragrant.

3. In a large bowl, toss together the sprouts, onion, chickpeas, and cranberries. Add the Lemon Vinaigrette and toss to coat. Serve immediately. To store extra salad, put the dressing and vegetables in separate airtight containers in the refrigerator for up to 2 days.

Serves 4 / Per Serving Calories: 343   Total fat: 13.8g   Saturated fat: 1.9g   Protein: 13.1g   Carbohydrates: 46.5g   Fiber: 12.8g   Cholesterol: 0mg

Quinoa Salad with Cannellini Beans, Tomatoes, and Lemon Vinaigrette

VEGETARIAN   VEGAN   GLUTEN-FREE

Prep time: 10 minutes   **Cooking time:** 20 minutes

Quinoa contains more protein than any other grain, making it an ideal base for this take-along lunch salad. The fluffy cooked quinoa grains soak up the lemony dressing as the salad sits, so if you make it in the morning, or even the night before, it will be that much more delicious by the time you're ready for lunch.

- 3 cups cooked quinoa (see Cooking Tip)
- ½ cup Lemon Vinaigrette (page 215)
- 1 (15-ounce) can cannellini beans, rinsed and drained
- 3 medium tomatoes, diced

1. In a large bowl, combine the quinoa and the Lemon Vinaigrette and toss to mix. Add the beans and tomatoes and toss to combine well.

2. Serve immediately, or store in the refrigerator in an airtight container for up to 2 days.

Serves 6 / Per Serving Calories: 393   Total fat: 7.2g   Saturated fat: 1g   Protein: 21.3g   Carbohydrates: 63.6g   Fiber: 20.5g   Cholesterol: 0mg

> **COOKING TIP**
>
> When you cook quinoa, measure the quinoa to water in a 1:2 ratio. Bring to a boil over medium-high heat. Reduce the heat to low, cover, and cook for 15 to 20 minutes, until the quinoa is tender. Set aside off the heat, covered, for 5 minutes. Transfer to a large flat bowl and cool to room temperature.

Brown Rice and Black Bean Salad with Spinach and Lemon Vinaigrette

VEGETARIAN   VEGAN   DAIRY-FREE

Prep time: 10 minutes   **Cooking time:** 40 minutes

Combining brown rice and cooked beans makes this dish a complete protein. The tangy Lemon Vinaigrette and fresh spinach leaves make it a refreshing salad that's perfect for packing in a workday lunchbox. Brown rice takes a while to cook, so you might want to double the amount (use 2 cups uncooked rice to 4 cups water) so you'll have extra cooked rice for another dish.

- 1 cup brown rice
- 1 (15-ounce) can black beans, rinsed and drained
- 1 medium cucumber, peeled, halved lengthwise, and cut into slices
- 2 cups gently packed fresh spinach leaves
- 1 pint cherry tomatoes, halved
- ½ cup Lemon Vinaigrette (page 215)

1. To cook the rice, combine it with 2 cups of cold water in a medium lidded saucepan and bring to a boil. Reduce the heat to low, cover, and simmer for 35 to 40 minutes, until the liquid has been absorbed and the rice is tender. Transfer the cooked rice to a large bowl and let cool.

2. Add the beans, cucumber, spinach, tomatoes, and Lemon Vinaigrette. Toss to combine well. Store covered in the refrigerator for up to 1 day.

Serves 6 / Per Serving Calories: 424   Total fat: 7g   Saturated fat: 1.1g   Protein: 19g   Carbohydrates: 74.1g   Fiber: 13.2g   Cholesterol: 0mg

Shrimp Salad over Greens with Yogurt Dressing

GLUTEN-FREE

Prep time: 5 minutes   **Cooking time:** None

Succulent shrimp top fresh lettuce, ripe cherry tomatoes, and crunchy cucumber, all drizzled with a tangy yogurt dressing. This dish is everything you want in a salad: crisp, refreshing, flavorful, and full of protein. Throw in a few diced red or yellow bell pepper or sliced scallions for even more pizazz.

- 12 ounces broiled or grilled shrimp (see Grilled Shrimp Tacos, page 152)
- 1 tablespoon freshly squeezed lemon juice
- 2 tablespoons olive oil
- 1 head butter or Bibb lettuce, torn into bite-size pieces
- 1 small cucumber, diced
- 8 to 10 cherry tomatoes, halved
- ½ cup Yogurt Dressing (page 216)

1. In a medium bowl, toss the shrimp with the lemon juice and the olive oil.

2. In a large bowl, add the lettuce, cucumber, and tomatoes and toss to mix. Divide the salad mixture among four serving plates. Top each salad with one-quarter of the shrimp and then drizzle the Yogurt Dressing over the top.

Serves 4 / Per Serving Calories: 301   Total fat: 18.9g   Saturated fat: 4g   Protein: 21.5g   Carbohydrates: 9.5g   Fiber 4.3g   Cholesterol: 179mg

> **ON-THE-GO TIP**
>
> This salad makes a great take-along lunch. First, divide the dressing among four jars. Next add the shrimp, then the cucumbers, avocado, and lettuce. Cap the jars and refrigerate. Take one jar along with you. When you're ready to eat, pour the contents of the jar out into a serving bowl, toss, and enjoy.

Spinach Salad with Chicken and Sun-Dried Tomatoes and Basil Vinaigrette

GLUTEN-FREE   DAIRY-FREE

Prep time: 10 minutes   **Cooking time:** None

This simple salad is a tasty way to turn leftover roasted chicken into a hearty and satisfying lunch. The sweet-tart balsamic vinegar–based dressing gets intense flavor from sun-dried tomatoes and chopped fresh basil. Cherry tomatoes in the salad add a fresh tomatoey note that plays well with the dried tomatoes in the dressing.

½ cup Balsamic Vinaigrette (page 214)
2 halves sun-dried tomato (packed in oil, drained), minced
1 tablespoon minced fresh basil
6 cups gently packed fresh spinach leaves
1 cup cherry tomatoes
2 cups (about 10 ounces) shredded cooked chicken breast (see Roasted Chicken with Vegetables, page 166)

1. In a small bowl, whisk together the Balsamic Vinaigrette, sun-dried tomatoes, and basil.

2. In a large bowl, toss the spinach and cherry tomatoes.

3. Add the chicken and the vinaigrette and toss to coat. Serve immediately. To store, cover and put in the refrigerator until ready to eat, up to 6 hours. If you wish to store the salad longer, keep the spinach and cherry tomatoes, the chicken, and the vinaigrette in separate containers in the refrigerator and toss together before serving.

Serves 4 / Per Serving Calories: 336   Total fat: 19.6g   Saturated fat: 2.4g   Protein: 30.6g   Carbohydrates: 10.9g   Fiber: 3.3g   Cholesterol: 73mg

Garden Salad with Chicken and Balsamic Vinaigrette

GLUTEN-FREE   DAIRY-FREE

Prep time: 10 minutes   **Cooking time:** 6 minutes

This simple salad is quick to make and extremely satisfying. Fresh lettuce, cooked chicken, tomatoes, and avocado are dressed in a sweet-tangy Balsamic Vinaigrette. It's a convenient meal to take with you to work or school and a delicious use of leftover cooked chicken.

- 1 head butter or Bibb lettuce, torn into bite-size pieces
- ½ cup Balsamic Vinaigrette (page 214)
- 2 medium tomatoes, chopped
- 1 ripe avocado, diced
- 2 cups (about 10 ounces) diced cooked chicken breast (see Roasted Chicken with Vegetables, page 166)

1. In a large bowl, toss together the lettuce and most of the vinaigrette, reserving about 2 tablespoons.

2. To serve, divide the dressed lettuce among four serving plates. Arrange the tomatoes, avocado, and chicken on top of the lettuce, dividing equally. Drizzle with the reserved vinaigrette. Serve immediately.

Serves 4 / Per Serving Calories: 355   Total fat: 22.1g   Saturated fat: 3.1g   Protein: 29.6g   Carbohydrates: 12.2g   Fiber: 5.1g   Cholesterol: 73mg

> **ON-THE-GO TIP**
>
> This salad makes a great take-along lunch. To make it commute-friendly, pack the salad ingredients into pint-size mason jars with the vinaigrette on the bottom and the lettuce on top. Just pour the contents of the jar out into a serving bowl, toss, and enjoy.

Roasted Vegetable Pitas with Pesto Mayonnaise

VEGETARIAN

Prep time: 5 minutes   **Cooking time:** None

The rich sweetness of caramelized roasted vegetables pairs wonderfully with tangy goat cheese. A quick spread that combines Homemade Mayonnaise and Fresh Basil Pesto adds even more flavor. Feel free to substitute whole-grain sandwich bread for the pita if you prefer.

- ¼ cup Homemade Mayonnaise (page 217)
- 1 tablespoon Fresh Basil Pesto (page 219)
- 2 whole-wheat pitas, halved
- 2 cups roasted vegetables, left over from Balsamic-Roasted Vegetables with Quinoa (page 139)
- ½ cup (2 ounces) crumbled goat cheese
- 4 lettuce leaves, such as butter or Bibb

1. In a small bowl, stir together the mayonnaise and pesto.

2. Spread the mayonnaise mixture into the pita halves, dividing equally. Fill each pita half with ½ cup of the roasted vegetables, 2 tablespoons of the goat cheese, and a large lettuce leaf. Serve immediately, or wrap and refrigerate until ready to serve, up to 6 hours.

Serves 4 / Per Serving Calories: 244   Total fat: 12.6g   Saturated fat: 4.7g   Protein: 9.2g   Carbohydrates: 25.5g   Fiber: 3.5g   Cholesterol: 20mg

Egg Salad Sandwich with Greek Yogurt and Dill

VEGETARIAN

Prep time: 10 minutes   **Cooking time:** None

Because Greek yogurt is substituted for most of the mayonnaise, this egg salad is considerably lighter than most. The yogurt also adds a welcome tang and pairs beautifully with the dill.

8 hard-boiled eggs, chopped
⅔ cup plain Greek yogurt
1 tablespoon Homemade Mayonnaise (page 217)
1 teaspoon dried dill
¾ teaspoon salt
½ teaspoon freshly ground black pepper
8 slices whole-grain bread
2 cups fresh spinach leaves
2 tomatoes, thinly sliced

1. In a large bowl, combine the eggs and yogurt and stir with a fork, mashing the eggs as you mix. Add the mayonnaise, dill, salt, and pepper and stir to combine.

2. Arrange four of the bread slices on your work surface. Spoon on the egg mixture equally among them, flattening with the back of a fork. Top each sandwich with ½ cup of the spinach and a few of the tomato slices. Place the remaining four bread slices on top and slice each sandwich on the diagonal. Serve immediately, or wrap the sandwiches individually and refrigerate until ready to serve, up to 1 day. If you wish to make them farther in advance, keep the egg salad, bread, and vegetables separate in the refrigerator and assemble the sandwiches just before serving or in the morning on the day you plan to eat them.

Serves 4 / Per Serving Calories: 367   Total fat: 12g   Saturated fat: 3.6g   Protein: 24.2g   Carbohydrates: 38.3g   Fiber: 11g   Cholesterol: 330mg

Curried Chicken Salad Lettuce Wraps with Homemade Mayonnaise

DAIRY-FREE

Prep time: 10 minutes   **Cooking time:** None

Curry powder gives a spicy kick to this quick chicken salad, which is made with leftover cooked chicken. Chunks of crisp apple add a satisfying textural contrast and a bit of sweetness to temper the heat. The chicken salad is made with a quick Homemade Mayonnaise. You can use any crisp red or green apple.

- 2½ cups (about 12 ounces) chopped cooked chicken breast (see Roasted Chicken with Vegetables, page 166)
- 1 large apple, cored and diced
- ½ cup Homemade Mayonnaise (page 217)
- 1 tablespoon curry powder
- ¾ teaspoon salt
- ½ teaspoon freshly ground black pepper
- 4 large lettuce leaves, such as butter or Bibb

1. In a medium bowl, combine the chicken and apple. Add the mayonnaise and stir to combine. Add the curry powder, salt, and pepper and stir to mix well. Taste and adjust seasoning as needed.

2. Arrange the lettuce leaves on your work surface and divide the chicken mixture evenly among them, piling the mixture in a line down the center of each leaf. Wrap the lettuce around the filling like a burrito. Wrap well in plastic wrap and store in the refrigerator until ready to eat, up to 1 day.

Serves 4 / Per Serving Calories: 289   Total fat: 13.1g   Saturated fat: 1.5g   Protein: 27.8g   Carbohydrates: 15.8g   Fiber: 1.9g   Cholesterol: 81mg

Spiced Chicken Wraps with Yogurt Dressing and Fresh Mint

Prep time: 10 minutes   **Cooking time:** None

Using delicious leftover Tandoori-Spiced Chicken Breast and tangy Yogurt Dressing from previous meals makes these flavorful wraps as easy to make as PB&J. Be sure to check tortilla labels carefully to choose a brand that does not contain preservatives and other additives. If you can't find suitable tortillas, you can make these wraps using large lettuce leaves instead.

- 4 whole-wheat tortillas
- 2 cups (about 10 ounces) cooked sliced Tandoori-Spiced Chicken Breast (page 170)
- ½ cup Yogurt Dressing (page 216)
- ½ small cucumber, cut in thin slices
- ¼ cup chopped fresh mint leaves
- 1 small jalapeño pepper, seeded and thinly sliced (optional)

1. Lay the four tortillas on your work surface. Put the chicken down the center of the tortillas, dividing it equally among them. Top each with 2 tablespoons of the dressing, one-quarter of the cucumber slices, 1 tablespoon of the mint, and a few jalapeño pepper slices (if using).

2. Wrap up the tortillas burrito-style and serve immediately, or wrap tightly in plastic wrap and refrigerate until ready to serve, up to 1 day.

Serves 4 / Per Serving Calories: 251   Total fat: 7.9g   Saturated fat: 2.4g   Protein: 29.4g   Carbohydrates: 14.5g   Fiber 2.2g   Cholesterol: 78mg

Korean Pork Lettuce Wraps with Fresh Herbs

DAIRY-FREE

Prep time: 10 minutes   **Cooking time:** None

Lettuce wraps aren't some new-fangled invention precipitated by the rise in popularity of gluten-free and grain-free diets. Lettuce has been traditionally used as a wrapper for savory fillings all over Asia. In Korea, bulgogi, *or marinated and grilled meat, is often served with a platter of lettuce leaves, fresh herbs, and other vegetables so diners can make their own lettuce wraps at the table.*

- 16 ounces stir-fried cubed pork
- 8 large lettuce leaves, such as butter or Bibb
- 1 cup grated carrot
- 1 cup grated cucumber
- ½ cup fresh mint leaves
- ½ cup fresh basil leaves
- Chili paste (optional)

1. Lay the lettuce leaves on a work surface and fill them with the pork, dividing the meat equally. Top each with 2 tablespoons each of carrot and cucumber, a few mint leaves, a few basil leaves, and a dollop of chili paste (if using).

2. Wrap the lettuce leaves up burrito-style and serve, or wrap them individually and refrigerate until ready to serve, up to 1 day.

Serves 4 / Per Serving Calories: 185   Total fat: 4.1g   Saturated fat: 1.4g   Protein: 30.6g   Carbohydrates: 5g   Fiber: 1.8g   Cholesterol: 83mg

Smoky Red Lentil Soup with Greens

VEGETARIAN   VEGAN   GLUTEN-FREE   DAIRY-FREE

Prep time: 10 minutes   **Cooking time:** 45 minutes

Red lentils make a beautifully red-hued soup. Quick cooking and full of fiber, lentils are an excellent and inexpensive source of vegetarian protein. This spicy soup gets better with time, so make it a day or two ahead if you are able, or make a double batch and eat leftovers all week. Don't be tempted to skip the splash of lemon juice at the end since it really brings the flavors together.

1 tablespoon olive oil
1 medium onion, diced
2 garlic cloves, minced
2 teaspoons ground cumin
2 teaspoons smoked paprika
1 teaspoon ground turmeric
1 teaspoon salt
¼ teaspoon ground cinnamon
2 medium carrots, peeled and sliced
7 cups vegetable broth
1½ cups dry red lentils
1 (14.5-ounce) can diced tomatoes with their juice
4 cups gently packed fresh spinach leaves
Juice of 1 freshly squeezed lemon

1. In a large stockpot over medium-high heat, heat the olive oil and add the onions and garlic. Sauté, stirring frequently, until the onions have softened, about 5 minutes.

2. Add the cumin, paprika, turmeric, salt, and cinnamon and cook, stirring, for 1 minute.

3. Add the carrots, vegetable broth, lentils, and tomatoes and bring to a boil. Reduce the heat to medium-low and simmer for 30 to 35 minutes, uncovered, until the lentils are soft. Stir in the spinach and cook until wilted, about 2 minutes.

4. Just before serving, stir in the lemon juice. Serve hot. To store, let the soup come to room temperature, put in airtight containers, and refrigerate for up to 5 days. The soup can also be frozen for up to 3 months. Reheat before serving.

Serves 4 / Per Serving Calories: 413 Total fat: 7.3g Saturated fat: 1.4g Protein: 29.9g Carbohydrates: 57.6g Fiber: 26g Cholesterol: 0mg

> **ON-THE-GO TIP**
>
> If you prefer not to use a microwave, get a good thermos and pack hot soup into it in the morning to take with you to work or school.

Spicy Black Bean Soup with Vegetables

VEGETARIAN VEGAN GLUTEN-FREE DAIRY-FREE

Prep time: 10 minutes   **Cooking time:** 30 minutes

Black beans make a rich, dark, brothy soup that is just the thing to warm you up on a cold day. This version is full of vegetables—carrots, sweet potatoes, and green beans—making it super nutritious and very satisfying. Jalapeño peppers give it a bit of a spicy kick. If you like your food spicier, add more jalapeño peppers, or leave them out if you prefer a milder flavor.

- 2 tablespoons olive oil
- 1 medium onion, diced
- 2 garlic cloves, minced
- 1 to 3 jalapeño peppers, seeded and diced
- 4 medium carrots, sliced
- 1 large sweet potato, peeled and cut into ½-inch cubes
- 2 cups fresh or frozen green beans
- 1 teaspoon cayenne pepper
- 2 teaspoons chili powder
- 2 teaspoons ground cumin
- 2 teaspoons salt
- 4 cups vegetable broth
- 2 (15-ounce) cans black beans, rinsed and drained

1. In a large stockpot, heat the olive oil over medium-high heat. Add the onion and cook, stirring, until softened, about 5 minutes. Add the garlic and cook for 30 seconds more. Add the jalapeño pepper, carrots, sweet potato, green beans, cayenne pepper, chili powder, cumin, and salt and cook, stirring occasionally, for 2 to 3 minutes. Add the broth and black beans and bring to a boil. Reduce the heat to medium-low and simmer, uncovered, for 20 minutes, until the vegetables are tender.

2. Serve hot. Leftovers can be stored, covered, in the refrigerator for up to 1 week or in the freezer for up to 3 months. For the meal plan, freeze half of the soup in individual servings for Week Three.

Serves 8 / Per Serving Calories: 333   Total fat: 5.8g   Saturated fat: 1g   Protein: 17.2g   Carbohydrates: 54.7g   Fiber: 13.3g   Cholesterol: 0mg

> ON-THE-GO TIP
>
> If you prefer not to use a microwave oven, get a good thermos and pack hot soup into it in the morning to take with you to work or school.

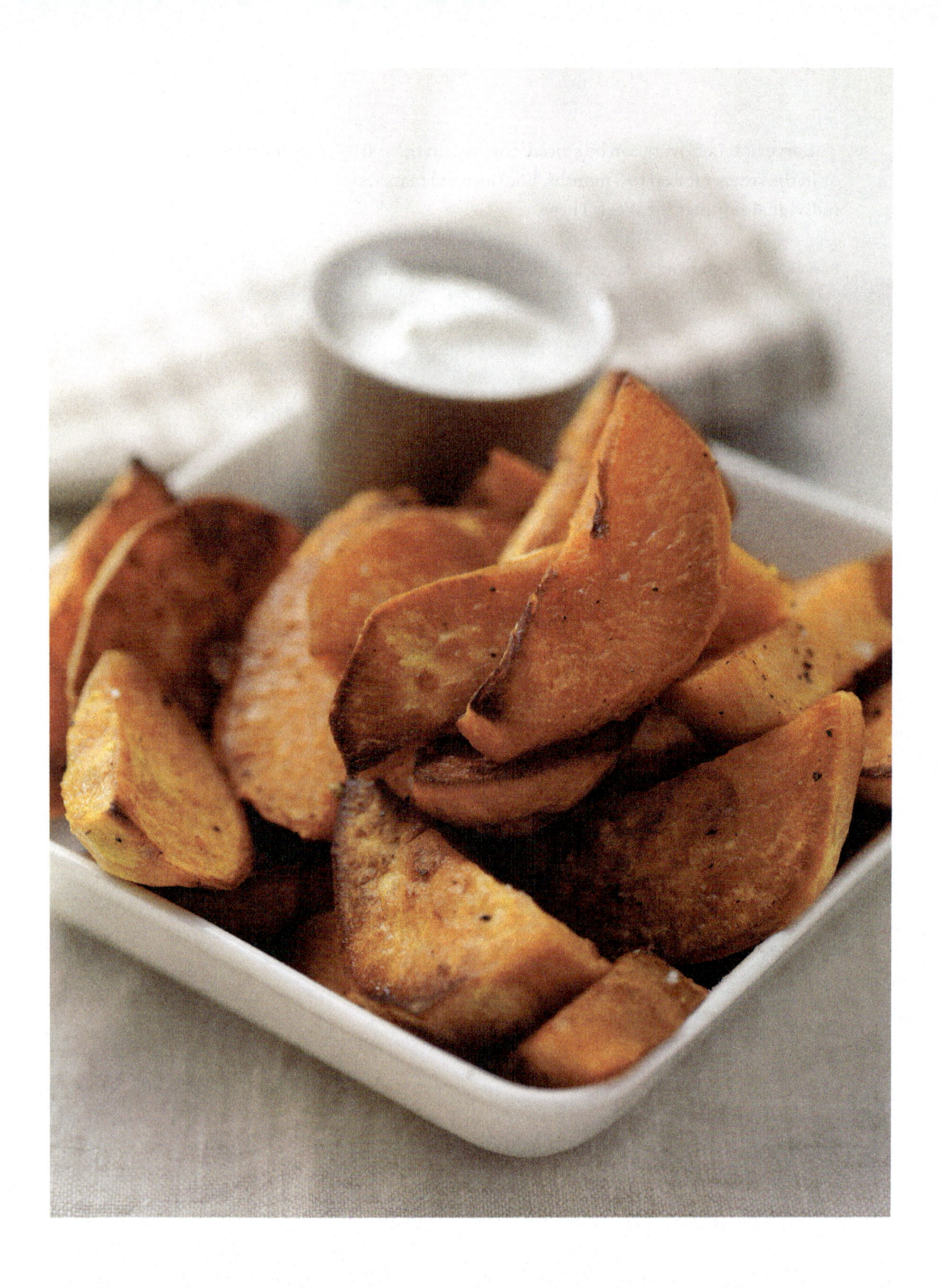

6

Snacks

Pineapple Coconut Trail Mix   112
Peanut Butter Energy Bites   113
Tropical Sweet Bars   114
Apple Walnut Bars   115
Banana Nut Bread   116
Honey Sesame Crackers   118
Creamy Peanut Butter–Yogurt Dip   119
Spiced Roasted Chickpeas   120
Smoky-Sweet Chili Almonds   121
Basil Garlic Zucchini Chips   122
Oven-Baked Sweet Potato Fries   123
Pesto White Bean Spread   124

Pineapple Coconut Trail Mix

VEGETARIAN   VEGAN   GLUTEN-FREE   DAIRY-FREE

Prep time: 2 minutes   **Cooking time:** None

Sweet-and-nutty trail mix makes a great snack anytime, but is particularly great to have on hand when you're out and about. Pop a bagful into your purse or backpack, and you'll be ready whenever hunger strikes.

- 1½ cups whole almonds
- 1 cup diced unsweetened dried pineapple
- ½ cup unsweetened shredded coconut

Put the almonds, pineapple, and coconut in a big jar or storage container and shake to mix. Store in an airtight container at room temperature for up to 3 months.

Makes 3 cups (six ½-cup servings) / **Per Serving** Calories: 175   Total fat: 14.1g   Saturated fat: 2.9g   Protein: 5.4g   Carbohydrates: 9.7g   Fiber: 4g   Cholesterol: 0mg

Peanut Butter Energy Bites

VEGETARIAN   VEGAN   GLUTEN-FREE   DAIRY-FREE

Prep time: 10 minutes (plus 30 minutes to chill dough)   **Cooking time:** None

These nutty nibbles taste like cookies but are so much more nutritious. You can enjoy them guilt-free for an energy-boosting snack anytime of day, or even for a healthful breakfast. They've got the protein and fiber you need to get going in the morning, and they are the perfect complement to a cup of herbal tea. Feel free to substitute other nut butters for the peanut butter.

- 1 cup old-fashioned rolled oats
- ⅔ cup unsweetened shredded coconut
- ½ cup all-natural peanut butter
- ½ cup ground flaxseed
- ⅓ cup honey
- 1 teaspoon vanilla extract

1. In a medium bowl, combine the oats, coconut, peanut butter, flaxseed, honey, and vanilla, and stir to mix thoroughly. Refrigerate for 30 minutes.

2. Roll the chilled dough into balls about the size of a walnut. Store in the refrigerator in an airtight container for up to 1 week.

Makes about 24 bites (about 12 servings) / Per Serving Calories: 159   Total fat: 8.8g   Saturated fat: 2.7g   Protein: 4.6g   Carbohydrates: 16.6g   Fiber: 3g   Cholesterol: 0mg

INGREDIENT VARIATIONS

The variation possibilities of these energy bites are virtually endless. You could substitute other nut butters—like almond, cashew, or hazelnut—for the peanut butter. You could use maple syrup instead of honey. Or try adding dried fruits, chopped nuts, or even chocolate chips if you like.

Tropical Sweet Bars

VEGETARIAN   VEGAN   GLUTEN-FREE   DAIRY-FREE

Prep time: 5 minutes (plus 5 minutes to soak the pineapple and 20 minutes to chill)
Cooking time: None

Surprisingly sweet, dried pineapple delivers a big dose of natural sugar in addition to its complex tropical fruit flavor. Here it's combined with rich cashews and chewy shredded coconut for easy-to-make bars that will give you energy and keep you going strong throughout the day.

- 2 cups unsweetened dried pineapple
- ⅔ cup hot water
- 2 cups cashews
- ½ cup unsweetened shredded coconut
- ¼ teaspoon salt

1. Line an 8-inch square baking pan with parchment paper.

2. Put the pineapple in a small bowl and cover with the hot water. Let soak for about 5 minutes and then drain, discarding the soaking liquid.

3. In the bowl of a food processor (or blender), add the pineapple, cashews, coconut, and salt and process until finely ground and a sticky batter forms.

4. Transfer the mixture into the prepared baking pan and press it down with your hands (wetting them first will prevent sticking), until it is even and firmly packed. Freeze for 10 to 15 minutes, until firm. Cut into 16 bars and serve immediately. To store, put in an airtight container and refrigerate for up to 1 week.

Makes 16 bars / Per Serving Calories: 176   Total fat: 13.6g   Saturated fat: 4.8g   Protein: 4g   Carbohydrates: 12.2g   Fiber: 1.9g   Cholesterol: 0mg

Apple Walnut Bars

VEGETARIAN   VEGAN   GLUTEN-FREE   DAIRY-FREE

Prep time: 15 minutes   **Cooking time:** 35 minutes

Packed full of toasted walnuts, apples, and oats and flavored with a hint of cinnamon, these bars are make a great after-school snack. They're also perfect for packing in your bag and taking to work.

- 2 cups chopped walnuts
- 2 cups old-fashioned rolled oats
- 1½ cups (about 8 ounces) pitted and halved dates
- 2 teaspoons ground cinnamon
- ¼ teaspoon salt
- 2 apples, such as Fuji, cored and chopped

1. Preheat the oven to 350°F. Line a large baking sheet with parchment paper and line an 8-inch square baking pan with parchment paper, leaving enough paper hanging over the edge so you can lift the bars out of the pan.

2. Spread the walnuts and oats on the prepared baking sheet in a thin layer. Toast them in the oven for 10 to 15 minutes, until they become fragrant.

3. Transfer the toasted walnuts and oats to a food processor (or blender). Add the dates, cinnamon, and salt. Process until the mixture resembles a coarse, crumbly meal. Add the apple and pulse until it is finely chopped. Continue processing until the mixture is smooth and begins to stick together.

4. Pour the mixture into the prepared baking pan, and press it into a compact layer using your hands (it helps to wet them first) or a spatula.

5. Bake for 20 minutes. Let the bars cool in the pan for about 10 minutes. Use the parchment paper to lift the bars out of the pan. Cut into 12 bars and serve immediately, or store in the refrigerator in an airtight container for up to 1 week.

Makes 12 bars / Per Serving Calories: 250   Total fat: 13.2g   Saturated fat: 0.9g   Protein: 7.3g   Carbohydrates: 30g   Fiber: 5.2g   Cholesterol: 0mg

Banana Nut Bread

VEGETARIAN   DAIRY-FREE

Prep time: 10 minutes   **Cooking time:** 50 minutes

Sweetened with honey and full of banana flavor, you won't be able to tell that this version of banana bread is made with whole-wheat flour instead of white flour. Walnuts add a good crunch and a hint of cinnamon adds spice. Bake up a loaf and you'll have easy-to-grab, healthful snacks for days. For a bit of extra sweetness and added texture, add ½ cup of raisins along with the walnuts, if desired.

¼ cup coconut oil, melted, plus more for the pan
1½ cups whole-wheat flour
1¼ teaspoons baking powder
½ teaspoon baking soda
½ teaspoon ground cinnamon
Pinch of salt
2 egg whites, lightly beaten
3 medium ripe bananas, mashed
½ cup honey
½ cup chopped walnuts

1. Preheat the oven to 350°F. Lightly coat an 8-by-4-inch loaf pan with coconut oil.

2. In a medium bowl, stir together the flour, baking powder, baking soda, cinnamon, and salt.

3. In a large bowl, mix together the egg whites, bananas, honey, and the ¼ cup melted coconut oil until well combined. Add the flour mixture to the egg mixture and stir just until combined. Gently fold in the walnuts. Spoon the batter into the prepared loaf pan and spread to make an even layer.

4. Bake 45 to 50 minutes, or until golden brown and a toothpick inserted in the center comes out clean. Let cool in the pan for 10 to 15 minutes before slicing. Serve warm or at room temperature. Store leftovers in an airtight container at room temperature for up to 1 week. Leftovers can also be wrapped and frozen for up to 3 months. Bring to room temperature before serving.

Makes 12 slices / Per Serving Calories: 188 Total fat: 7.8g Saturated fat: 4.2g Protein: 3.8g Carbohydrates: 27.5g Fiber: 1.7g Cholesterol: 0mg

Honey Sesame Crackers

VEGETARIAN   GLUTEN-FREE   DAIRY-FREE

Prep time: 5 minutes (plus 20 minutes to cool)   **Cooking time:** 2 minutes

Made with three ingredients that are likely in your pantry already, these little crackers are nutty, crunchy, and addictive. They make a great snack when you're craving a little something sweet.

3 tablespoons coconut oil, plus more for the pan
1 cup honey
1 cup sesame seeds

1. Line a baking sheet with aluminum foil and coat it lightly with coconut oil.

2. In a small saucepan, bring the honey and coconut oil to a boil over medium-high heat, stirring constantly. Cook, stirring, until the honey begins to brown, about 2 minutes.

3. Remove from the heat and stir in the sesame seeds. Pour the mixture onto the prepared baking sheet and let the mixture cool for about 20 minutes. Break the crackers into about 12 pieces. Store them between layers of parchment paper in an airtight container in the refrigerator for up to 1 week.

Makes about 12 crackers / Per Serving Calories: 184   Total fat: 9.4g   Saturated fat: 3.8g   Protein: 2.2g   Carbohydrates: 26.1g   Fiber: 1.5g   Cholesterol: 0mg

Creamy Peanut Butter–Yogurt Dip

VEGETARIAN GLUTEN-FREE

Prep time: 2 minutes   **Cooking time:** None

This creamy peanut butter–flavored dip is a delicious addition to apple or pear wedges, bananas, celery sticks, or just about anything else you can think of to dunk in it. It uses only three ingredients, two of which are likely in your pantry at all times, so it's easy to whip up on a moment's notice.

- 1 cup plain yogurt
- ¼ cup all-natural peanut butter
- 1½ tablespoons honey

In a small bowl, stir the yogurt, peanut butter, and honey together until smooth. Serve immediately, or store in the refrigerator in an airtight container for up to 1 week.

Serves 4 / Per Serving Calories: 160   Total fat: 8.9g   Saturated fat: 2.3g   Protein: 7.5g   Carbohydrates: 13.3g   Fiber: 1g   Cholesterol: 4mg

Spiced Roasted Chickpeas

VEGETARIAN   VEGAN   GLUTEN-FREE   DAIRY-FREE

Prep time: 5 minutes   **Cooking time:** 30 to 40 minutes

These spicy, crunchy nibbles are perfect to snack on when the afternoon drags at work. They've got the protein you need to get you through the afternoon and the fiber to keep you feeling full all the way until dinner. It's simple to make a large batch, and they keep well in an airtight container in your pantry.

- 2 (15-ounce) cans chickpeas, rinsed and drained
- 2 tablespoons cooking oil
- 1 teaspoon ground cumin
- 1 teaspoon chili powder
- ½ teaspoon cayenne pepper
- ½ teaspoon salt

1. Preheat the oven to 400°F. Line a large baking sheet with parchment paper.

2. In a large bowl, add the chickpeas, cooking oil, cumin, chili powder, cayenne pepper, and salt and toss until well coated.

3. Spread the chickpeas in the prepared baking sheet in an even layer. Bake for 30 to 40 minutes, until crisp. Serve immediately, or cool to room temperature and store in an airtight container at room temperature for up to 1 week.

Makes 16 servings / Per Serving Calories: 210   Total fat: 5g   Saturated fat: 0.6g
Protein: 10.3g   Carbohydrates: 32.4g   Fiber: 9.3g   Cholesterol: 0mg

---

INGREDIENT VARIATIONS

Roasted chickpeas are a blank slate that works with many different flavor combinations. Try curry powder, smoked paprika, lemon or lime, or whatever else strikes your fancy. You could even do a sweet version with 2 tablespoons of coconut sugar mixed with 1 teaspoon of ground cinnamon.

Smoky-Sweet Chili Almonds

VEGETARIAN   GLUTEN-FREE   DAIRY-FREE

Prep time: 5 minutes (plus 5 minutes to drain the almonds)   **Cooking time:** 55 minutes

Plain roasted almonds are delicious, but sometimes you crave an alternative with a bit more bite. So give this spiced version a whirl. With a distinctive smoky flavor from smoked paprika and a hint of chili powder, they're as addictive as store-bought smoked almonds.

- Coconut oil, for the pan
- 1 egg white
- 1 tablespoon water
- 3 cups almonds
- ½ cup honey
- 1 tablespoon salt
- 1 teaspoon smoked paprika
- 1 teaspoon ground cumin
- ½ teaspoon chili powder

1. Preheat the oven to 300°F. Lightly coat a large baking sheet with coconut oil.

2. In a large bowl, whisk together the egg white and water until foamy. Stir in the almonds. Put the almonds in a colander and let drain for 5 minutes.

3. In a large bowl, add the almonds, honey, salt, paprika, cumin, and chili powder and toss to coat. Spread the mixture in an even layer in the prepared baking sheet.

4. Bake for 15 minutes. Stir the almond mixture around and spread it out again in an even layer. Reduce the heat to 275°F and bake for 40 minutes more, stirring several times. Remove the pan from the oven and let the almonds cool for several minutes before breaking the clusters apart. Serve immediately, or cool completely and store in an airtight container at room temperature for up to 2 weeks.

Makes 12 servings / Per Serving Calories: 183   Total fat: 12g   Saturated fat: 0.9g   Protein: 5.4g   Carbohydrates: 17g   Fiber: 3.1g   Cholesterol: 0mg

Basil Garlic Zucchini Chips

VEGETARIAN   VEGAN   GLUTEN-FREE   DAIRY-FREE

Prep time: 10 minutes   **Cook time:** 2 to 3 hours

These crispy, salty, garlicky, herby chips satisfy that late-afternoon junk food craving with aplomb. You can eat them on their own or try dipping them in your favorite yogurt- or sour cream–based dip. Parmesan cheese, cayenne pepper, ground cumin, or smoked paprika would all create wonderfully addictive flavors. Sprinkle any cheese, dried spices, or fresh herbs on just after taking them out of the oven. Don't be tempted to slice the zucchini too thin or they'll burn. About $1/16$ inch—about the width of a nickel—is the ideal thickness.

- 2 tablespoons cooking oil
- 1 garlic clove, minced
- 4 medium zucchini (long and thin), cut in very thin slices
- ¼ cup minced fresh basil
- 1 teaspoon salt

1. Preheat the oven to your oven's lowest temperature setting (150°F to 200°F, if possible), and line two large baking sheets with parchment paper.

2. In a small bowl, mix the oil and garlic together.

3. Brush the parchment paper in the pans lightly with the garlic-oil mixture. Arrange the zucchini slices in a single layer in the prepared pans, and brush the tops lightly with the garlic-oil mixture.

4. Bake the zucchini slices for 2 to 3 hours, until very crisp (if cooking at a higher temperature, reduce the cooking time). Remove from the oven and sprinkle immediately with the basil and salt. Let cool on the baking sheet, and then transfer to an airtight container and store at room temperature for up to 3 days.

Serves 4 / Per Serving Calories: 93   Total fat: 7.2g   Saturated fat: 1.1g   Protein: 2.5g   Carbohydrates: 6.9g   Fiber: 2.2g   Cholesterol: 0mg

Oven-Baked Sweet Potato Fries

VEGETARIAN   VEGAN   GLUTEN-FREE   DAIRY-FREE

Prep time: 10 minutes   **Cooking time:** 30 minutes

When you're craving French fries, this spiced sweet potato version is sure to surprise you. Even though they're oven baked, they crisp up beautifully and deliver the salty crunch you want in a fry. Serve them with Romesco Sauce (page 220) or Homemade Mayonnaise (page 217) if you're feeling really decadent.

- 3 large sweet potatoes, peeled and cut into ¼-inch-wide sticks
- 3 tablespoons olive oil
- 2 tablespoons coconut sugar
- 1 tablespoon salt
- 2 teaspoons chili powder
- 1 teaspoon ground cumin

1. Preheat the oven to 450°F. Line a large baking sheet with parchment paper.

2. In a large bowl, toss the sweet potato sticks with the oil. Add the coconut sugar, salt, chili powder, and cumin and toss to mix well.

3. Transfer the sweet potatoes to the prepared baking sheet and spread them out in an even layer. Bake for 15 minutes. Flip the fries and return the pan to the oven to bake for another 10 to 15 minutes, until browned and crisp. Let cool for a few minutes before serving.

Serves 6 / Per Serving Calories: 256   Total fat: 7.5g   Saturated fat: 1.1g   Protein: 2.5g   Carbohydrates: 46.4g   Fiber: 6.5g   Cholesterol: 0mg

Pesto White Bean Spread

VEGETARIAN   VEGAN   GLUTEN-FREE   DAIRY-FREE

Prep time: 5 minutes   **Cooking time:** None

Creamy white beans mixed with Fresh Basil Pesto and a splash of lemon juice make a divine dip or spread for crudités, whole-wheat pita triangles, or grain-free crackers. The beans themselves are rather humble, but they make an ideal backdrop for the fresh herbs and citrus.

- 1 (15-ounce) can cannellini beans, rinsed and drained
- 2 tablespoons freshly squeezed lemon juice
- 2 tablespoons Fresh Basil Pesto (page 219)
- 2 tablespoons olive oil
- ½ teaspoon salt
- 2 tablespoons water

In the bowl of a food processor (or blender), add the beans, lemon juice, Fresh Basil Pesto, olive oil, and salt and process to a thick paste. Add the water and process to combine thoroughly. If the mixture is too thick, add a bit more water. Serve immediately, or store in the refrigerator in an airtight container for up to 5 days.

Makes about 2 cups (eight ¼-cup servings) / Per Serving Calories: 208   Total fat: 4g   Saturated fat: 0.6g   Protein: 12.6g   Carbohydrates: 32g   Fiber: 13.3g   Cholesterol: 0mg

INGREDIENT TIP

If you don't have Fresh Basil Pesto on hand, you can substitute either a store-bought pesto (just be sure to check the ingredients for additives) or you can use 2 tablespoons minced fresh basil combined with 2 minced garlic cloves.

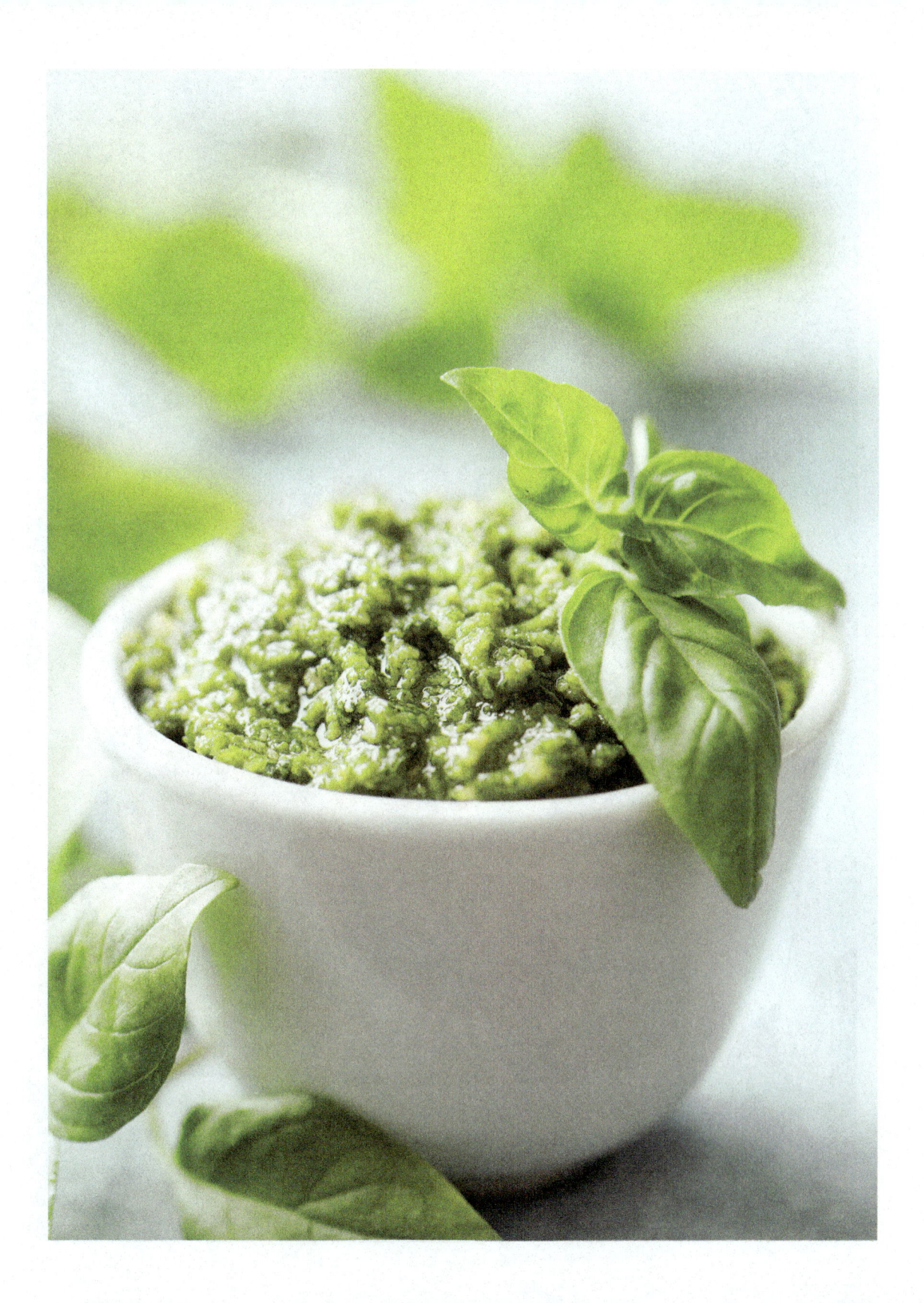

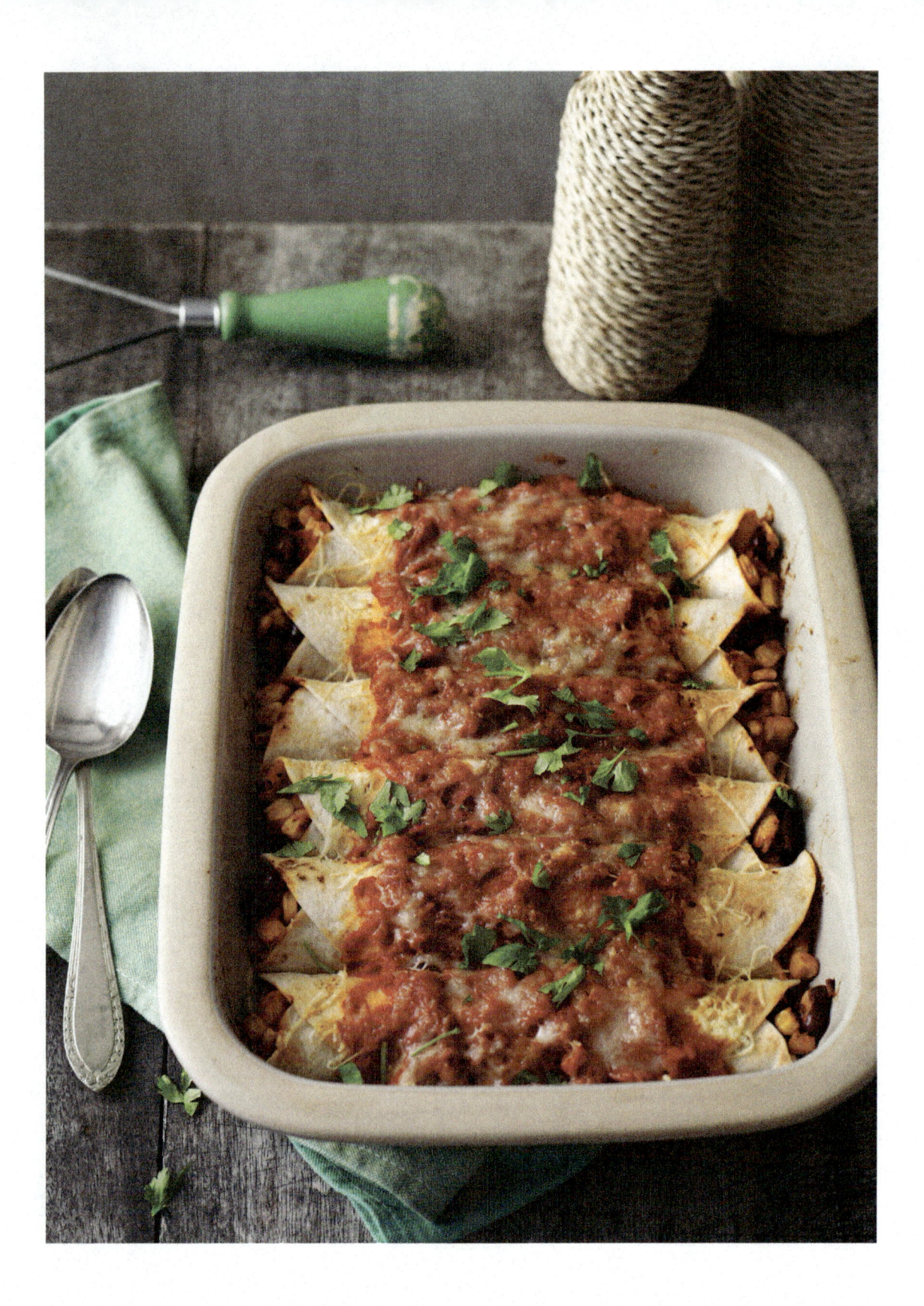

Vegetarian Dinners

Stacked Eggplant Parmesan   128
Vegetarian Chili with Pinto Beans   130
Pumpkin and Chickpea Curry   132
Chickpea Tostadas with Cashew Cheese   133
Spinach and White Bean Enchiladas with Cashew Cheese   135
Roasted Butternut Squash and Black Bean Burritos with Goat Cheese   137
Balsamic-Roasted Vegetables with Quinoa   139
Quinoa-Stuffed Peppers with Black Beans and Yogurt Dressing   141
Whole-Wheat Pasta with Chickpeas and Spicy Tomato Sauce   143
Vegetable Stew   144
Risotto with Mushrooms and Peas   146
Brussels Sprouts Hash with Caramelized Onions and Poached Eggs   148

Stacked Eggplant Parmesan

VEGETARIAN GLUTEN-FREE

Prep time: 10 minutes   **Cooking time:** 30 minutes

Succulent eggplant slices layered with Spicy Tomato Sauce and creamy fresh mozzarella is comfort food at its best. Almond flour stands in for the traditional bread crumbs, and adds a nutty richness to the coating that actually improves on the original. A crisp green salad would round out this meal perfectly.

- 1½ cups Spicy Tomato Sauce (page 221), plus ½ cup
- 1 egg, lightly beaten
- 2 cups almond flour
- 1 teaspoon salt
- ½ teaspoon freshly ground black pepper
- 2 tablespoons olive oil
- 2 medium eggplant, cut into ¼-inch-thick slices
- 2 ounces fresh mozzarella, thinly sliced, plus 2 ounces

1. Preheat the oven to 350°F. Spoon ½ cup of the Spicy Tomato Sauce into the bottom of an 8-by-11-inch baking dish, spreading it to evenly coat the bottom of the dish.

2. Put the egg in a shallow bowl. In a separate shallow bowl, stir together the almond flour, salt, and pepper.

3. In a large skillet, heat the olive oil over medium-high heat. Dip each slice of eggplant first into the egg and then into the almond flour mixture. Add the coated eggplant to the skillet a few slices at a time (don't crowd) and cook until browned, about 3 minutes per side. Put the eggplant slices on a paper towel-lined plate to drain.

4. Place a single layer of the eggplant slices on the bottom of the prepared baking dish. Top with 2 ounces of the mozzarella, and then add another layer of eggplant slices. Pour the remaining 1½ cups of sauce over and around the eggplant slices. Top with the remaining 2 ounces of mozzarella.

5. Bake for about 15 minutes, until the sauce is bubbly and the cheese is melted and beginning to brown.

Serves 4 / Per Serving Calories: 355   Total fat: 19.1g   Saturated fat: 6.9g   Protein: 24.9g   Carbohydrates: 27.6g   Fiber 12.8g   Cholesterol: 71mg

> COOKING TIP
>
> Eggplant can sometimes have a bitter edge to it. You can remove this bitterness by salting the eggplant before cooking it. Salt the eggplant slices generously on both sides and set them on a double layer of paper towels or a clean dishtowel to drain for 15 minutes. Rinse the salt off and pat the slices very dry with paper towels or a clean dishtowel.

Vegetarian Chili with Pinto Beans

VEGETARIAN   VEGAN   GLUTEN-FREE   DAIRY-FREE

Prep time: 10 minutes   **Cooking time:** 55 minutes

This hearty pinto bean chili has all the flavors of the classic meat-based version, but without the meat. Packed with veggies and beans—and redolent with chiles and spices—it cooks much more quickly than the traditional version as well. Top it with your favorite garnishes—try Guacamole (page 212), Cashew Cheese (page 224), Salsa Verde (page 218), store-bought hot or mild tomato salsa, plain yogurt or sour cream, shredded cheese, diced onions, or chopped fresh cilantro.

- 1 tablespoon olive oil
- 1 medium onion, diced
- 3 garlic cloves, minced
- 2 red bell peppers, seeded, deribbed, and diced
- 2 medium carrots, diced
- 2 to 3 jalapeño peppers, seeded and minced
- 1 tablespoon chili powder
- 2 teaspoons smoked paprika
- 1 teaspoon salt
- ¾ teaspoon cayenne pepper
- 1 (6-ounce) can tomato paste
- 2 (15-ounce) cans pinto beans
- 1 (28-ounce) can diced tomatoes with their juice

1. In a Dutch oven or stockpot set over medium-high heat, heat the olive oil. Add the onion and cook for about 5 minutes, stirring frequently, until softened. Add the garlic, carrots, and bell peppers and continue to cook, stirring frequently, for about 3 minutes. Add the jalapeño peppers, chili powder, paprika, salt, cayenne pepper, and tomato paste and cook, stirring, for 1 minute.

2. Add the pinto beans and the tomatoes, stir, and bring to a boil. Reduce the heat to medium-low and simmer for about 45 minutes, uncovered, until the liquid has thickened and the pinto beans are tender. Serve hot. Store in the refrigerator in an airtight container for up to 5 days or in the freezer for up to 3 months.

....

Serves 8 / Per Serving Calories: 447   Total fat: 3.7g   Saturated fat: 0.6g   Protein: 25.4g   Carbohydrates: 80.2g   Fiber 20.4g   Cholesterol: 0mg

Pumpkin and Chickpea Curry

VEGETARIAN   VEGAN   GLUTEN-FREE   DAIRY-FREE

Prep time: 10 minutes   **Cooking time:** 20 minutes

Bright-orange, sweet-fleshed pumpkin makes a stunning and equally delicious curry. The sweet pumpkin mingles beautifully with the hot curry and cayenne pepper. Serve this curry over brown rice or quinoa.

- 1 tablespoon olive oil
- 1 small onion, thinly sliced
- 4 cups diced pumpkin (1 medium pumpkin)
- 1 tablespoon curry powder
- 1 teaspoon salt
- ½ teaspoon cayenne pepper
- ½ cup vegetable broth
- 1 (15-ounce) can chickpeas, rinsed and drained
- 1 (14.5-ounce) can diced tomatoes with their juice

1. Heat the oil in a large skillet over medium-high heat. Add the onion and cook for about 3 minutes, stirring, until the onion begins to soften.

2. Reduce the heat to medium, and add the pumpkin, curry powder, salt, and cayenne pepper, and cook for 1 minute, stirring. Stir in the broth, chickpeas, and tomatoes and bring to a boil.

3. Cover, reduce the heat to low, and simmer for about 20 minutes, until the vegetables are tender.

Serves 4 / Per Serving Calories: 539   Total fat: 10.9g   Saturated fat: 1.6g   Protein: 25g   Carbohydrates: 90.4g   Fiber 27.4g   Cholesterol: 0mg

INGREDIENT TIP

Substitute any winter squash for the pumpkin. Butternut squash can often be found diced in bags (frozen or fresh) and is a great time-saver.

Chickpea Tostadas with Cashew Cheese

VEGETARIAN   VEGAN   GLUTEN-FREE   DAIRY-FREE

Preparation time: 10 minutes   **Cooking time:** 20 minutes

A crispy corn tortilla base is topped with creamy cashew cheese, crunchy roasted chickpeas, lettuce, and salsa for a fantastic vegetarian and dairy-free take on this Mexican classic. Use any kind of salsa you like to give this dish your own spin. For even more flavor, top it with chopped fresh cilantro, diced onions or sliced scallions, and a squeeze of lime.

Olive oil

2 tablespoons low-sodium soy sauce

1 tablespoon freshly squeezed lime juice

2 teaspoons chili powder

1 teaspoon cayenne pepper

1 teaspoon salt

1 teaspoon freshly ground black pepper

1 teaspoon ground cumin

1 teaspoon smoked paprika

1 (15-ounce) can chickpeas, rinsed and drained

8 corn tortillas

1 cup Cashew Cheese (page 224)

2 cups shredded lettuce

1 cup salsa

1. Preheat the oven to 400°F. Line two large baking sheets with aluminum foil and lightly coat with olive oil.

2. In a medium bowl, stir together the soy sauce, lime juice, chili powder, cayenne pepper, salt, black pepper, cumin, and smoked paprika. Add the chickpeas and toss to coat well. ▶

Vegetarian Dinners

Chickpea Tostadas with Cashew Cheese, continued

3. Spread the chickpeas in a single layer on one of the prepared baking sheets, and bake in the preheated oven for about 18 minutes, tossing them once, until crisp and golden.

4. While the chickpeas are roasting, arrange the tortillas in a single layer on the other prepared baking sheet. Brush the tops of the tortillas lightly with olive oil. Bake the tortillas in the oven (you can do this while the chickpeas are roasting) for about 10 minutes, flipping them over once during cooking, until slightly crisp.

5. To assemble the tostadas: Spoon 1 tablespoon of Cashew Cheese onto each warm tortilla and spread it around. Top with some of the chickpeas, lettuce, and a generous scoop of salsa. Serve immediately. Store leftovers in separate containers for up to 1 week in the refrigerator.

Serves 6 / Per Serving Calories: 430   Total fat: 11.2g   Saturated fat: 1.7g   Protein: 20.2g   Carbohydrates: 66.9g   Fiber 16.5g   Cholesterol: 0mg

Spinach and White Bean Enchiladas with Cashew Cheese

VEGETARIAN   VEGAN   DAIRY-FREE

Prep time: 10 minutes   **Cooking time:** 30 minutes

Hearty spinach, corn, and bean–filled tortillas are bathed in a spicy red sauce that's quick to make and full of flavor. Top these with a dollop of Guacamole (page 212), sour cream or plain yogurt, or a sprinkling of sliced scallions or chopped fresh cilantro, if you like.

- 2 tablespoons olive oil, plus more for the pan
- 1 garlic clove, minced
- ¼ cup whole-wheat flour
- ¼ cup tomato paste
- 2 teaspoons ground cumin
- 2 teaspoons chili powder
- ½ teaspoon salt
- ¼ teaspoon freshly ground black pepper
- 3 cups vegetable broth
- 1 cup canned cannellini beans, rinsed and drained
- 1 cup frozen corn kernels
- 1 (10-ounce) package frozen chopped spinach, thawed and squeezed dry
- 8 corn tortillas
- 2 tablespoons chopped cilantro (optional)
- 1 cup Cashew Cheese (page 224)

1. Preheat the oven to 375°F. Lightly coat an 8-by-11-inch baking dish with olive oil.

2. To make the sauce, heat the olive oil in a medium saucepan over medium heat. Add the garlic, flour, tomato paste, cumin, chili powder, salt, and pepper and cook, whisking constantly, for 1 minute. Whisk in the vegetable broth and bring the mixture to a boil. Reduce the heat to low and simmer about 8 minutes, stirring occasionally, until the sauce thickens. ▶

Spinach and White Bean Enchiladas with Cashew Cheese, continued

3. Meanwhile, in a large bowl, combine the beans, corn, and spinach.

4. To assemble the enchiladas, spread a few spoonfuls of the sauce in the bottom of the prepared baking dish.

5. Fill the tortillas with the spinach-corn-bean mixture, dividing equally, and roll them up into cylinders. Place the cylinders, seam-side down, in the baking dish. Cover with the remaining sauce.

6. Bake for about 20 minutes, until the tortillas are golden brown. Just before serving, drizzle the Cashew Cheese over the enchiladas (if the cheese is too thick, warm it a bit in a double boiler set over boiling water) and top with cilantro, if desired. Serve hot.

Serves 4 / Per Serving Calories: 494   Total fat: 16.2g   Saturated fat: 2.8g   Protein: 21.2g   Carbohydrates: 62.8g   Fiber 17.5g   Cholesterol: 0mg

Roasted Butternut Squash and Black Bean Burritos with Goat Cheese

VEGETARIAN

Prep time: 10 minutes **Cooking time:** 15 minutes

The caramelized sweetness of roasted butternut squash, spicy kick of jalapeño peppers, and creamy tang of goat cheese are a match made in heaven. This recipe uses butternut squash that you've preroasted along with canned black beans, so it's super quick to put this together on a busy evening. The burritos keep well, too, so pack up any leftovers to take for lunch or have for another dinner if you like.

Olive oil, for the pan
1½ cups roasted butternut squash (halve the recipe in prep ahead, page 44)
1 to 2 jalapeño peppers, seeded and diced
1 teaspoon ground cumin
1 teaspoon chili powder
1 teaspoon salt
½ teaspoon freshly ground black pepper
1 cup canned black beans, rinsed and drained
1 cup (4 ounces) goat cheese
Olive oil, for the pan
4 whole-wheat tortillas

1. Preheat the oven to 375°F. Lightly coat an 8-inch baking dish with olive oil. Wrap the tortillas in aluminum foil and warm in the oven while it heats up.

2. In a large bowl, combine the butternut squash, jalapeño peppers, cumin, chili powder, salt, and pepper and stir to combine well. Stir in the beans. ➤

Vegetarian Dinners

Roasted Butternut Squash and Black Bean Burritos with Goat Cheese, continued

3. Lay the warm tortillas on your work surface. Spoon about ⅓ cup of the vegetable mixture down the center of each tortilla. Top with the goat cheese, dividing it equally among the four tortillas. Fold the ends of the tortillas over the filling to keep it inside and then roll the burritos up into cylinders. Place the burritos, seam-side down, in the prepared baking dish.

4. Bake for about 15 minutes, until the tortillas are golden brown. Serve hot or let cool to room temperature, wrap individually, and refrigerate until ready to serve. Heat leftover burritos for about 15 minutes in a 375°F oven (or quickly in a microwave) before serving.

Serves 4 / Per Serving Calories: 374   Total fat: 11.8g   Saturated fat: 7.3g   Protein: 21.2g   Carbohydrates: 48.5g   Fiber 10.3g   Cholesterol: 10mg

Balsamic-Roasted Vegetables with Quinoa

VEGETARIAN   GLUTEN-FREE

Prep time: 10 minutes   **Cooking time:** 40 minutes

Roasting vegetables at high heat caramelizes their exteriors without drying out the interior. The resulting complex, slightly sweet vegetables are succulent and tender. Here mushrooms, bell peppers, zucchini, and red onion are roasted to moist, tender perfection in a balsamic marinade and then served over quinoa that soaks up all the flavors. A crumble of feta cheese adds richness and a bit of tang to cut the sweetness of the veggies.

- 2 tablespoons olive oil, plus more for the pan
- 2½ cups quinoa
- 8 ounces button or cremini mushrooms, halved or quartered if large
- 2 small zucchini, diced
- 1 red or yellow bell pepper, seeded, deribbed, and cut into strips
- ½ red onion, cut into small wedges
- 1 teaspoon salt
- ¼ teaspoon freshly ground black pepper
- 1 garlic clove, minced
- 3 tablespoons balsamic vinegar
- 1 cup (about 4 ounces) crumbled feta cheese

1. Preheat the oven to 425°F. Lightly coat a large baking sheet with olive oil.

2. In a large saucepan over medium-high heat, put 5 cups of water, stir in the quinoa, and bring to a boil. Cover, reduce the heat to medium-low, and cook for 15 to 20 minutes, until the quinoa is tender. Set aside off the heat, covered, for 5 minutes. Transfer 3 cups of the cooked quinoa to a storage container and refrigerate for later use. ▶

Vegetarian Dinners

Balsamic-Roasted Vegetables with Quinoa, continued

3. Meanwhile, on the prepared baking sheet, mix together the mushrooms, zucchini, bell pepper, and onion. In a small bowl, add the 2 tablespoons of oil with the salt, pepper, garlic, and vinegar and stir to mix. Drizzle the oil mixture over the vegetables and toss to coat. Spread out the vegetables in an even layer.

4. Roast for about 20 minutes, until the vegetables are tender. Transfer half of the vegetables to a storage container and refrigerate for future use.

5. To serve, mound ½ cup of the cooked quinoa on each of four plates. Top with a scoop of the roasted vegetables. Crumble the feta cheese over the top and serve immediately.

Serves 4 (plus extra servings of quinoa and veggies for other meals this week) /
Per Serving Calories: 275 Total fat: 12g Saturated fat: 5g Protein: 10.9g
Carbohydrates: 31g Fiber 3.9g Cholesterol: 25mg

Quinoa-Stuffed Peppers with Black Beans and Yogurt Dressing

VEGETARIAN GLUTEN-FREE

Prep time: 15 minutes   **Cooking time:** 1 hour and 10 minutes

As the grain that packs the highest protein punch, quinoa is ideal for vegetarian meals. Here it's combined with black beans and spices; baked inside fresh, sweet red bell peppers; and topped with a tangy yogurt dressing. These take a while to cook, but since the quinoa and Yogurt Dressing are both premade, the hands-on time is negligible. These stuffed peppers freeze well, so consider making a double batch and freezing the leftovers for a quick dinner in the future.

- 1 tablespoon olive oil
- ½ medium onion, finely chopped
- 2 garlic cloves, minced
- 1 (10-ounce) package frozen chopped spinach, thawed and squeezed dry
- 1 (14.5-ounce) can diced tomatoes, drained, juice reserved
- 1 tablespoon ground cumin
- 1 cup cooked quinoa (see Cooking Tip, page 96)
- 1 cup canned black beans, rinsed and drained
- 2 large red bell peppers, seeded, deribbed, and cut in half lengthwise
- ¾ cup Yogurt Dressing (page 216)

1. Preheat the oven to 350°F.

2. In a medium skillet, heat the olive oil over medium-high heat. Add the onion and cook for about 5 minutes, stirring frequently, until softened. Stir in the garlic and cook for about 1 minute. Add the spinach, tomatoes, and cumin and cook for about 5 minutes more, until most of the liquid has evaporated. Remove from the heat and stir in the cooked quinoa and beans. ▶

Quinoa-Stuffed Peppers with Black Beans and Yogurt Dressing, continued

3. Pour the reserved tomato juice into an 8-by-8-inch baking dish and arrange the pepper halves, cut-side up, in a single layer. Fill each half with the quinoa mixture, dividing the mixture evenly among the peppers.

4. Cover the baking dish with aluminum foil and bake for about 45 minutes, until the peppers are tender. Uncover the baking dish and bake for 15 minutes more, or until the filling is nicely browned. Let rest for 5 minutes in the baking dish. Then transfer the peppers to serving plates and drizzle with the Yogurt Dressing. Serve immediately.

Serves 4 (plus leftover quinoa for 2 future meals) / **Per Serving** Calories: 432   Total fat: 8.2g   Saturated fat: 1.6g   Protein: 22.2g   Carbohydrates: 69.7g   Fiber 14g   Cholesterol: 0mg

> **TIP TO DOUBLE AND FREEZE THIS RECIPE**
>
> This recipe is easily doubled by simply doubling the quantities listed for the filling and peppers and proceeding with the instructions as written. Yogurt dressing is best made within a few days of serving and should be refrigerated, not frozen. You'll need to be sure to cook an extra ½ cup of raw quinoa (for an extra 1 cup of cooked quinoa) when you do your prep ahead. To freeze the stuffed peppers, wrap them individually and store in the freezer for up to 3 months. Defrost in the refrigerator overnight, unwrap, and heat in a 350°F oven for about 20 to 30 minutes before serving.

Whole-Wheat Pasta with Chickpeas and Spicy Tomato Sauce

VEGETARIAN

Prep time: 5 minutes   **Cooking time:** 15 minutes

If you've got a batch of Spicy Tomato Sauce in your refrigerator or freezer, making this dinner is as easy as the old standby of pasta with jarred tomato sauce, but healthier and far more delicious. Chickpeas are an excellent source of low-fat, vegetarian protein and they add a nice bite to the sauce. Feel free to substitute another fresh herb, such as oregano or parsley, for the basil.

12 ounces whole-wheat pasta, such as penne or other short pasta
3 cups Spicy Tomato Sauce (page 221)
1 (15-ounce) can chickpeas, rinsed and drained
¼ cup chopped fresh basil
½ cup (2 ounces) crumbled feta cheese

1. Cook the pasta according to the package directions.

2. Meanwhile, heat the tomato sauce in a large saucepan over medium-high heat and bring to a boil. Add the chickpeas, reduce the heat to medium, and simmer for about 5 minutes until heated through.

3. Drain the pasta. Serve it topped with the sauce and sprinkled with the basil and the feta.

Serves 6 / Per Serving Calories: 469   Total fat: 9.1g   Saturated fat: 1.3g   Protein: 27.2g   Carbohydrates: 97.5g   Fiber: 23.4g   Cholesterol: 3mg

Vegetable Stew

VEGETARIAN   VEGAN   GLUTEN-FREE   DAIRY-FREE

Prep time: 15 minutes   **Cooking time:** 30 minutes

This recipe is only a guideline for the finished dish, because you can add any combination of vegetables and still have a delicious stew. The combination of vegetables in the ingredients provides an array of colors, textures, and tastes, giving you a complete culinary experience in one bowl. Eating many different colors of produce means you are getting a full range of antioxidants and nutrients, too.

1 teaspoon olive oil
1 small sweet onion, peeled and chopped
1 teaspoon minced garlic
½ teaspoon ground cumin
½ teaspoon ground coriander
1 large red bell pepper, seeded and chopped
2 carrots, peeled and chopped
2 cups vegetable broth
2 large tomatoes, chopped
½ cup canned cannellini beans, rinsed and drained
1 teaspoon fresh lemon juice
1 cup chopped kale
Freshly ground black pepper, to taste

1. In a large pot over medium heat, heat the oil and sauté the onion and garlic until softened, about 3 minutes.

2. Add the cumin and coriander and stir to coat, about 1 minute.

3. Add the red pepper and carrots and sauté for 5 minutes.

4. Stir in the vegetable broth, tomatoes, and cannellini beans.

5. Bring the stew to a boil and then reduce the heat to low.

6. Simmer the stew until the vegetables are tender, stirring often, about 15 to 17 minutes.

7. Add the lemon juice and kale, and heat until the kale is wilted, about 3 minutes.

8. Stir in the black pepper.

9. Serve hot.

....

Serves 4 / Per Serving Calories: 101   Total fat: 1.8g   Saturated fat: 0g   Protein: 4.4g   Carbohydrates: 17.7g   Fiber: 7.3g   Cholesterol: 0mg

Risotto with Mushrooms and Peas

VEGETARIAN   VEGAN   GLUTEN-FREE   DAIRY-FREE

Prep time: 10 minutes   **Cooking time:** 25 minutes

At its heart, risotto is just a humble rice dish, but many recipes make it seem rather intimidating to cook. In truth, cooking risotto is quite simple. The key steps are to stir the rice grains in hot oil to coat them before adding any liquid, and then to add hot liquid a little bit at a time, stirring constantly, until each addition is absorbed fully by the rice grains before adding the next. This version is, well, easy peasy.

4½ cups vegetable broth
1 tablespoon olive oil, plus 1 tablespoon
1 small onion, finely chopped
1 garlic clove, minced, plus 1 garlic clove, minced
1 cup Arborio rice
4 cups (12 ounces) thinly sliced button or cremini mushrooms
¾ cup frozen peas
¼ teaspoon freshly ground black pepper

1. In a medium saucepan set over medium-high heat, bring the broth to a simmer. Reduce the heat to low to keep the broth simmering.

2. In a large skillet over medium heat, heat 1 tablespoon of the olive oil. Add the onion and cook for 2 minutes, stirring frequently. Add 1 clove of garlic and cook for 30 seconds more, stirring frequently. Stir in the rice and cook for 1 minute while stirring to coat with the oil. Add ½ cup of the broth and cook for about 2 minutes, stirring frequently, until the liquid has absorbed. Stir in another ½ cup of the broth and cook for about 2 minutes more, stirring frequently, until the liquid has been absorbed. Continue adding the broth ½ cup at a time, stirring constantly after each addition, until the liquid is absorbed. This should take about 20 minutes.

3. In a large skillet over medium-high heat, heat the remaining 1 tablespoon olive oil. Add the mushrooms and cook for about 5 minutes, stirring occasionally, until the mushrooms are tender. Add the remaining 1 clove garlic and cook, stirring occasionally, for 1 minute. Remove from the heat.

4. Stir the mushrooms into the rice along with the peas and pepper. Cook for about 3 minutes more, until heated through. Serve immediately.

Serves 4 / Per Serving Calories: 390   Total fat: 9.2g   Saturated fat: 1.6g   Protein: 12.7g   Carbohydrates: 66.5g   Fiber 6.6g   Cholesterol: 0mg

Brussels Sprouts Hash with Caramelized Onions and Poached Eggs

VEGETARIAN   GLUTEN-FREE   DAIRY-FREE

Prep time: 5 minutes   **Cooking time:** 25 minutes

Eggs are too delicious and versatile to be reserved for breakfast. This savory egg-topped vegetable hash is a perfect example of why eggs are—or at least should be—perfect as a dinner food. The beauty of a perfectly poached egg here is that the runny yolk mingles with the veggie mixture below to make a rich and satisfying sauce.

- 2 tablespoons olive oil, plus 1 tablespoon
- 1 onion, thinly sliced
- ½ teaspoon salt, plus ½ teaspoon
- ¼ teaspoon freshly ground black pepper, plus ¼ teaspoon
- 2 tablespoons apple cider vinegar
- 1 tablespoon honey
- 1½ pounds Brussels sprouts, trimmed and thinly sliced
- 1 cup water
- 8 eggs

1. Set a medium saucepan of water over high heat and bring to a boil. Reduce the heat to low.

2. In a large skillet, heat 2 tablespoons of olive oil over medium heat. Add the onion, ½ teaspoon of the salt, and ¼ teaspoon of the pepper, and cook for about 10 minutes, stirring occasionally, until the onion is soft and golden brown. Stir in the vinegar and honey, and cook, stirring, for 3 minutes, until carmelized. Transfer the onion to a small bowl.

3. In the same skillet, heat the remaining 1 tablespoon olive oil over medium-high heat. Add the Brussels sprouts along with the remaining ½ teaspoon salt and ¼ teaspoon pepper. Cook for about 6 minutes, stirring occasionally, until the edges of the sprouts begin to brown. Add the water and cook for about 3 minutes, stirring occasionally, until the water has mostly evaporated and the Brussels sprouts are tender.

4. Meanwhile, carefully crack the eggs into the simmering water and cook for 4 minutes, until the whites are set but the yolks are still runny.

5. Stir the caramelized onions into the Brussels sprouts and cook for about 2 minutes until heated through. Serve the Brussels sprouts hash hot, topped with the eggs.

Serves 4 / Per Serving Calories: 348   Total fat: 19.9g   Saturated fat: 4.4g   Protein: 18.3g   Carbohydrates: 30.2g   Fiber 6.5g   Cholesterol: 327mg

COOKING TIP

The key to perfectly poached eggs is to drop the raw eggs into simmering, not boiling, water, and then immediately reduce the heat to low to keep the water at a steady simmer (do not let the water boil once the eggs are in). Crack the eggs into the water, one at a time, starting at 12 o'clock and move counter-clockwise. Set a timer for 4 minutes and remove the eggs promptly, starting with the one at 12 o'clock and moving clockwise, using a slotted spoon.

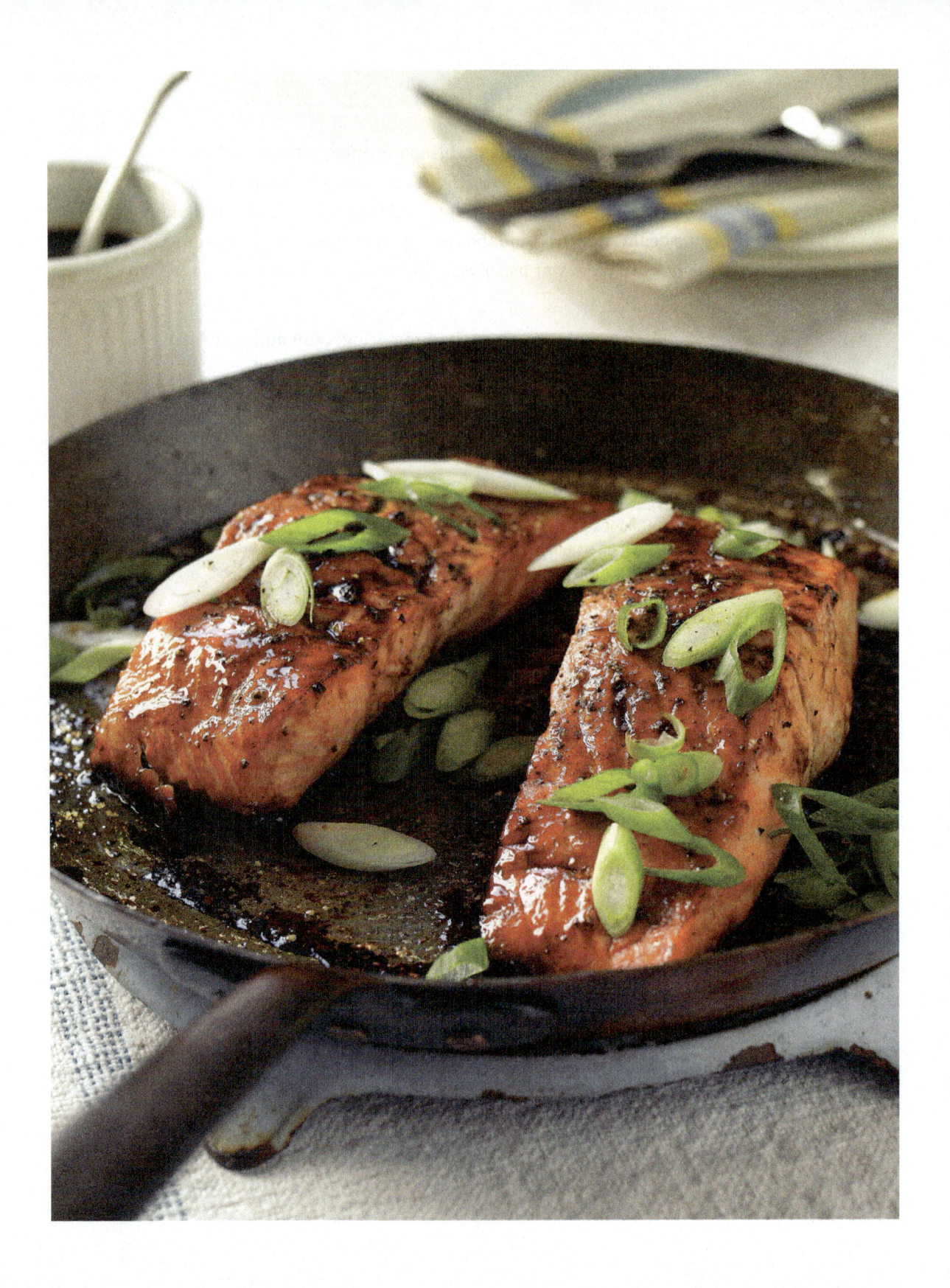

8

Fish and Seafood Dinners

Grilled Shrimp Tacos with Salsa Verde and Spicy Slaw   152
Garlic-Broiled Shrimp and Peppers over Quinoa   154
Seared Ahi Tuna with Chili-Lime Aioli   156
Balsamic-Glazed Wild Salmon with Garlicky Sautéed Spinach   157
Red Snapper with Spiced Pumpkin Seed Butter   159
Oven-Roasted Monkfish and Asparagus with Romesco Sauce   160
Soy-Glazed Cod with Japanese-Style Pickled Cucumber   161
Italian Fish Stew   163

Grilled Shrimp Tacos with Salsa Verde and Spicy Slaw

GLUTEN-FREE   DAIRY-FREE

Prep time: 10 minutes (plus 15 minutes to marinate the shrimp)   **Cooking time:** 6 minutes

Quick and easy to grill, shrimp make a flavorful and light taco filling. A short dunk in a spicy lime-based marinade is all they need to soak up the Mexican flavors. A few minutes on the grill kisses them with smoke. Layer the shrimp into warm soft corn tortillas and top with tangy Salsa Verde and crisp, spicy slaw for a divine meal that's ready in no time.

1 pound shrimp, peeled and deveined
½ teaspoon salt
Juice of 2 freshly squeezed limes
1 garlic clove, minced
½ teaspoon ground cumin
½ teaspoon chili powder
1 tablespoon cooking oil, plus 1 tablespoon, plus more for the grill
½ small head of green or red cabbage (about 14 ounces), cored and thinly sliced
½ medium red onion, thinly sliced
1 to 2 jalapeño peppers, seeded and minced
¼ cup chopped fresh cilantro
Salt
Freshly ground black pepper
8 soft corn tortillas
1 cup Salsa Verde (page 218)

1. Thread the shrimp onto metal skewers, put the skewers in a large baking dish, and season with the salt. In a small bowl, stir together one-half of the lime juice, the garlic, cumin, chili powder, and 1 tablespoon of the cooking oil. Drizzle the mixture over the shrimp and turn to coat well. Refrigerate for 15 minutes.

2. While the shrimp are marinating, make the slaw. In a large bowl, toss together the cabbage, onion, jalapeño pepper, cilantro, and the remaining lime juice. Add the remaining 1 tablespoon of cooking oil, season with salt and pepper, and toss well. Set aside.

3. Brush the grill grates with cooking oil and heat the grill to medium-high. Remove the shrimp skewers from the marinade, letting the excess drip off, and place on the grill. Cook the skewers undisturbed for 2 to 3 minutes, until the bottom begins to brown. Turn the skewers over and grill for about 2 minutes, until the second side is browned slightly and the shrimp are cooked through. Push the cooked shrimp off the skewers onto a plate.

4. Heat the tortillas on the grill, or one at a time in a medium frying pan over medium-high heat.

5. To make the tacos, divide the shrimp equally among the tortillas. Top with a spoonful or two of Salsa Verde and pile some of the slaw on top. Serve immediately.

Serves 4 / Per Serving Calories: 430   Total fat: 10.5g   Saturated fat: 1.9g   Protein: 30.1g   Carbohydrates: 30.7g   Fiber: 6g   Cholesterol: 239mg

INGREDIENT TIP

Peeling and deveining shrimp is time consuming, but you can find peeled and deveined shrimp in the freezer section of most supermarkets (just make sure what you buy is raw) or at any fish counter. To defrost frozen shrimp, either refrigerate overnight or set in a bowl of cold water for about 20 minutes. Drain and pat dry before proceeding with the recipe.

Garlic-Broiled Shrimp and Peppers over Quinoa

GLUTEN-FREE DAIRY-FREE

Prep time: 10 minutes   **Cooking time:** 20 minutes

Shrimp is low in calories, high in protein, and quick cooking, making it a favorite of health-conscious cooks. Here it's bathed in a garlicky oil mixture and then broiled along with red bell peppers to seal in the juices. The garlicky oil is then used to flavor precooked quinoa, rounding out this delicious meal.

- 2 tablespoons olive oil, plus more for the baking dish
- 2¼ pounds shrimp, peeled and deveined
- 2 red bell peppers, seeded, deribbed, and cut into 1½-inch triangles
- 4 garlic cloves, minced
- 2 teaspoons smoked paprika
- ¾ teaspoon cayenne pepper
- 1½ teaspoons salt
- ½ cup vegetable broth
- 2 cups cooked quinoa (see Cooking Tip, page 96)

1. Preheat the broiler to high. Lightly coat a large shallow baking dish with oil.

2. In a large bowl, add the shrimp, bell peppers, olive oil, garlic, smoked paprika, cayenne pepper, and salt and toss to coat. Transfer the shrimp mixture to the prepared baking dish and spread out in a single layer.

3. Cook for 8 minutes, then flip the shrimp mixture and cook for about 7 minutes more, until the shrimp are cooked through and the bell peppers are tender. Transfer about one-third of the shrimp to a storage container and refrigerate for later use. Transfer the remaining remaining shrimp and the bell peppers to a bowl using a slotted spoon.

4. Scrape the sauce and any browned bits from the baking dish into a medium saucepan and add the vegtetable broth. Bring to a boil over medium-high heat. Reduce the heat to medium, stir in the cooked quinoa, and cook until heated through, about 5 minutes.

5. To serve, mound the quinoa onto four serving plates and top with the shrimp and bell peppers. Serve immediately. Leftovers can be stored in the refrigerator, covered, for up to 3 days.

Serves 4 (with extra shrimp for another meal) **/ Per Serving** Calories: 465   Total fat: 12.1g   Saturated fat: 2.1g   Protein: 52g   Carbohydrates: 60.7g   Fiber: 8.3g   Cholesterol: 358mg

Seared Ahi Tuna with Chili-Lime Aioli

GLUTEN-FREE DAIRY-FREE

Prep time: 5 minutes (plus 10 minutes to marinate the fish)   **Cooking time:** 6 minutes

Ahi, or yellowfin, tuna melts in your mouth with a deliciously rich, meaty flavor. Briefly steeped in a lime and chili–spiked marinade, the tuna is then seared just until the outside is cooked but the center is still rare and succulent.

   3 tablespoons olive oil, plus 1 tablespoon
   2 tablespoons freshly squeezed lime juice
   1 jalapeño pepper, seeded and minced
   4 (6-ounce) ahi tuna steaks (about 1 inch thick)
   ½ teaspoon salt
   ⅓ cup Homemade Mayonnaise (page 217)

1. In a small bowl, whisk together 3 tablespoons of the olive oil, the lime juice, and jalapeño pepper.

2. Season the tuna steaks on both sides with salt and put them in a large, shallow baking dish. Pour most of the olive oil mixture over the fish, reserving about 1½ tablespoons of the marinade. Turn the tuna steaks to coat and marinate for about 10 minutes.

3. To make the aioli, add the Homemade Mayonnaise to the bowl with the reserved marinade and stir to mix.

4. In a large skillet, heat the remaining 1 tablespoon of olive oil over medium-high heat. Add the fish and sear for 2 to 3 minutes until browned on the bottom. Turn the fish over and sear on the second side for 2 to 3 minutes until browned on the bottom. The fish should still be pink in the center. Serve immediately, topped with the aioli mixture.

Serves 4 / Per Serving Calories: 498   Total fat: 29.8g   Saturated fat: 5.5g   Protein: 51.1g   Carbohydrates: 4.9g   Fiber: 0g   Cholesterol: 13.3mg

Balsamic-Glazed Wild Salmon with Garlicky Sautéed Spinach

GLUTEN-FREE   DAIRY-FREE

Prep time: 10 minutes   **Cooking time:** 12 minutes

In this simple recipe the salmon is seared over high heat and then braised in a flavorful sauce just until it cooks through, which keeps it moist and tender and full of flavor. Served over a bed of garlicky spinach it is an elegant yet deceptively easy meal.

- 2 teaspoons coconut oil, plus 1 teaspoon
- 1 pound fresh spinach leaves
- 1 garlic clove, minced
- 4 (6-ounce) wild salmon fillets
- 1 teaspoon salt
- ½ teaspoon freshly ground black pepper
- 1 tablespoon honey
- 3 tablespoons balsamic vinegar
- ½ teaspoon cayenne pepper

1. In a large skillet, heat 1 teaspoon of the coconut oil over medium-high heat. Add the spinach and garlic and cook for about 2 minutes, tossing, until all the spinach is wilted. Transfer the spinach to a serving platter.

2. Wipe out the skillet and heat the remaining 2 teaspoons coconut oil over medium-high heat. Season the salmon fillets on both sides with the salt and pepper. Sear the fish for about 2 minutes, until it is browned on the bottom; then flip and sear for 1 to 2 minutes, until the second side is browned.

3. Meanwhile, in a small bowl, add the honey, vinegar, and cayenne pepper and stir to combine. Add the vinegar mixture to the skillet with the fish, and simmer for about 5 minutes until the liquid is reduced and the fish is cooked through. ▶

Fish and Seafood Dinners

Balsamic-Glazed Wild Salmon with Garlicky Sautéed Spinach, continued

4. Transfer the salmon to the platter with the spinach, and drizzle the sauce over the top. Serve immediately.

Serves 4 / Per Serving Calories: 395   Total fat: 18.4g   Saturated fat: 3g   Protein: 39.3g   Carbohydrates: 16.8g   Fiber: 1.9g   Cholesterol: 104mg

> INGREDIENT TIP
>
> Wild salmon is preferred over farmed by clean eaters since it's less likely to contain toxic chemicals or to have been treated with additives such as food coloring. Wild salmon is also much leaner than farmed salmon, which means it is easy to overcook and turn dry. Searing it to seal in the juices and then braising it gently in liquid is a good way to keep it moist and flavorful.

Red Snapper with Spiced Pumpkin Seed Butter

GLUTEN-FREE

Prep time: 5 minutes **Cooking time:** 10 minutes

Roasted pumpkin seeds, or pepitas, *a common ingredient in certain Mexican cuisines, add nutty flavor and a bit of crunch to this simple pan-seared fish dish. If you don't have pumpkin seeds, you could substitute sunflower seeds, chopped pistachios, or pine nuts. Serve this dish with lightly sautéed spinach, oven-roasted broccoli, or a simple green salad.*

- 2 tablespoons hulled, unsalted, roasted pumpkin seeds (*pepitas*)
- 1 tablespoon butter, at room temperature
- ½ teaspoon freshly grated lime zest
- 2 tablespoons freshly squeezed lime juice
- ¼ teaspoon chili powder
- 1 tablespoon olive oil
- 4 (6-ounce) red snapper fillets
- ½ teaspoon salt
- ¼ teaspoon freshly ground black pepper

1. In a small bowl, stir together the pumpkin seeds, butter, lime zest, lime juice, and chili powder.

2. In a large skillet, heat the olive oil over medium heat. Season the fish on both sides with salt and pepper and cook for 2 to 4 minutes per side, until browned and just cooked through. Transfer the fish to a serving platter.

3. Reduce the heat under the skillet to medium, add the pumpkin seed–butter mixture to the pan, and cook, stirring, until the butter is melted. Drizzle the sauce over the fish and serve hot.

Serves 4 / Per Serving Calories: 298   Total fat: 11.3g   Saturated fat: 3.3g   Protein: 45.9g   Carbohydrates: 1.1g   Fiber: 0g   Cholesterol: 88mg

Oven-Roasted Monkfish and Asparagus with Romesco Sauce

GLUTEN-FREE DAIRY-FREE

Prep time: 5 minutes   **Cooking time:** 15 minutes

Monkfish is a meaty, succulent fish that takes to many different preparations. Here it is roasted alongside asparagus spears. While the fish and veggies are roasting, whip up the quick Romesco Sauce—a Spanish sauce made of roasted red bell peppers thickened with ground almonds and spiked with sherry vinegar.

1 pound asparagus, trimmed
1 tablespoon olive oil, plus 1 tablespoon
½ teaspoon salt, plus ¼ teaspoon
½ teaspoon freshly ground black pepper, plus ¼ teaspoon
4 (6-ounce) monkfish fillets (about 1½ inches thick)
Romesco Sauce (page 220)

1. Preheat the oven to 425°F.

2. Toss the asparagus in a large baking sheet with 1 tablespoon of the olive oil, ½ teaspoon of the salt, and ½ teaspoon of the pepper.

3. On a separate baking sheet, arrange the monkfish fillets in a single layer and drizzle the remaining 1 tablespoon of olive oil over the top. Season with the remaining ¼ teaspoon salt and ¼ teaspoon pepper.

4. Place both sheets in the oven at the same time (if they can't fit side by side, put the asparagus below the fish). Cook for about 15 minutes, until the asparagus is tender and the fish is cooked through and flakes easily with a fork.

5. Serve the monkfish on top of the asparagus with a dollop of Romesco Sauce on top. Any leftovers can be stored, covered, in the refrigerator for up to 2 days.

Serves 4 / Per Serving Calories: 355   Total fat: 17.3g   Saturated fat: 2.1g   Protein: 41.1g   Carbohydrates: 4.7g   Fiber: 2.5g   Cholesterol: 94mg

Soy-Glazed Cod with Japanese-Style Pickled Cucumber

DAIRY-FREE

Prep time: 5 minutes (plus 15 minutes to marinate the fish and 15 minutes to marinate the cucumbers)   **Cooking time:** 15 minutes

Cod, a delightfully meaty yet mild flavored fish, is well suited to many different preparations. Here it gets a glaze made from basic pantry ingredients—low-sodium soy sauce, honey, rice vinegar, and sesame oil—and a topping of quick pickles that add just the right crunchy-salty-sweet-tangy contrast to the fish. Serve with a side of steamed brown rice or soba (buckwheat) noodles tossed with a splash of sesame oil, if desired.

- 3 tablespoons low-sodium soy sauce, plus 1 tablespoon
- 2 tablespoons honey, plus 1 teaspoon
- ¼ cup rice vinegar, plus 1 tablespoon
- 1 tablespoon sesame oil, plus 1 teaspoon
- 1 tablespoon mirin or white wine
- Juice of 1 freshly squeezed lime
- 1 tablespoon peeled minced fresh ginger
- 2 garlic cloves, minced
- 4 (6-ounce) cod fillets
- 1 medium cucumber, peeled, halved lengthwise, seeded, and sliced thin
- 1 tablespoon sesame seeds

1. Preheat the oven to 400°F.

2. In a small bowl, stir together 3 tablespoons of the soy sauce, 2 tablespoons of the honey, 1 tablespoon of the rice vinegar, 1 tablespoon of the sesame oil, the mirin, lime juice, ginger, and garlic. Place the fish in a baking dish and pour the marinade over the top. Turn the fillets to thoroughly coat. Let the fish marinate at room temperature for about 15 minutes. ▶

Soy-Glazed Cod with Japanese-Style Pickled Cucumber, continued

3. To make the pickled cucumber, in a medium bowl, add the remaining 1 tablespoon soy sauce, 1 teaspoon honey, ¼ cup rice vinegar, and 1 teaspoon sesame oil and stir to combine. Add the cucumber slices and toss to coat. Let sit at room temperature for 10 to 15 minutes.

4. Remove the fish from the marinade, reserving the marinade, and place it in a clean baking dish. Roast for 12 to 15 minutes, turning once during cooking and brushing twice with the marinade, until the fish is cooked through and flakes easily with a fork.

5. Meanwhile, transfer the reserved marinade to a small saucepan and bring to a boil over high heat. Reduce the heat to low and cook for 5 to 7 minutes, stirring freuently, until the sauce thickens.

6. To serve, top each fish fillet with ¼ cup of the pickled cucumber and sprinkle with sesame seeds. Serve immediately.

Serves 4 / Per Serving Calories: 276 Total fat: 4.8g Saturated fat: 0.7g Protein: 27.5g Carbohydrates: 18.3g Fiber: 0.8g Cholesterol: 90mg

Italian Fish Stew

GLUTEN-FREE   DAIRY-FREE

Prep time: 5 minutes   **Cooking time:** 15 minutes

This is just the kind of stew you imagine Italian fisherman enjoying on their days off. Firm, succulent white fish is gently poached in a hearty, garlic-spiked, tomatoey broth. The firmer the fish, the better, so something like cod or halibut is your best bet.

- 2 tablespoons olive oil
- 1 small onion, thinly sliced
- 3 garlic cloves, minced
- 1 (28-ounce) can diced tomatoes with their juice
- ½ cup water
- 1 teaspoon salt
- 1 teaspoon dried oregano
- ½ teaspoon cayenne pepper
- 1 pound white fish (cod or halibut) fillets, cut into pieces

1. In a Dutch oven or stockpot, heat the olive oil over medium-high heat. Add the onion and cook for about 3 minutes, stirring frequently, until it begins to soften. Add the garlic and cook for 1 minute, stirring frequently. Add the tomatoes, water, salt, oregano, and cayenne pepper and bring to a simmer. Simmer for 5 minutes.

2. Add the fish, cover the pot, and simmer for about 5 minutes more, until the fish is cooked through. Serve hot.

Serves 4 / Per Serving Calories: 242   Total fat: 8.2g   Saturated fat: 1.2g   Protein: 28.4g   Carbohydrates: 13.3g   Fiber: 3.5g   Cholesterol: 13.3mg

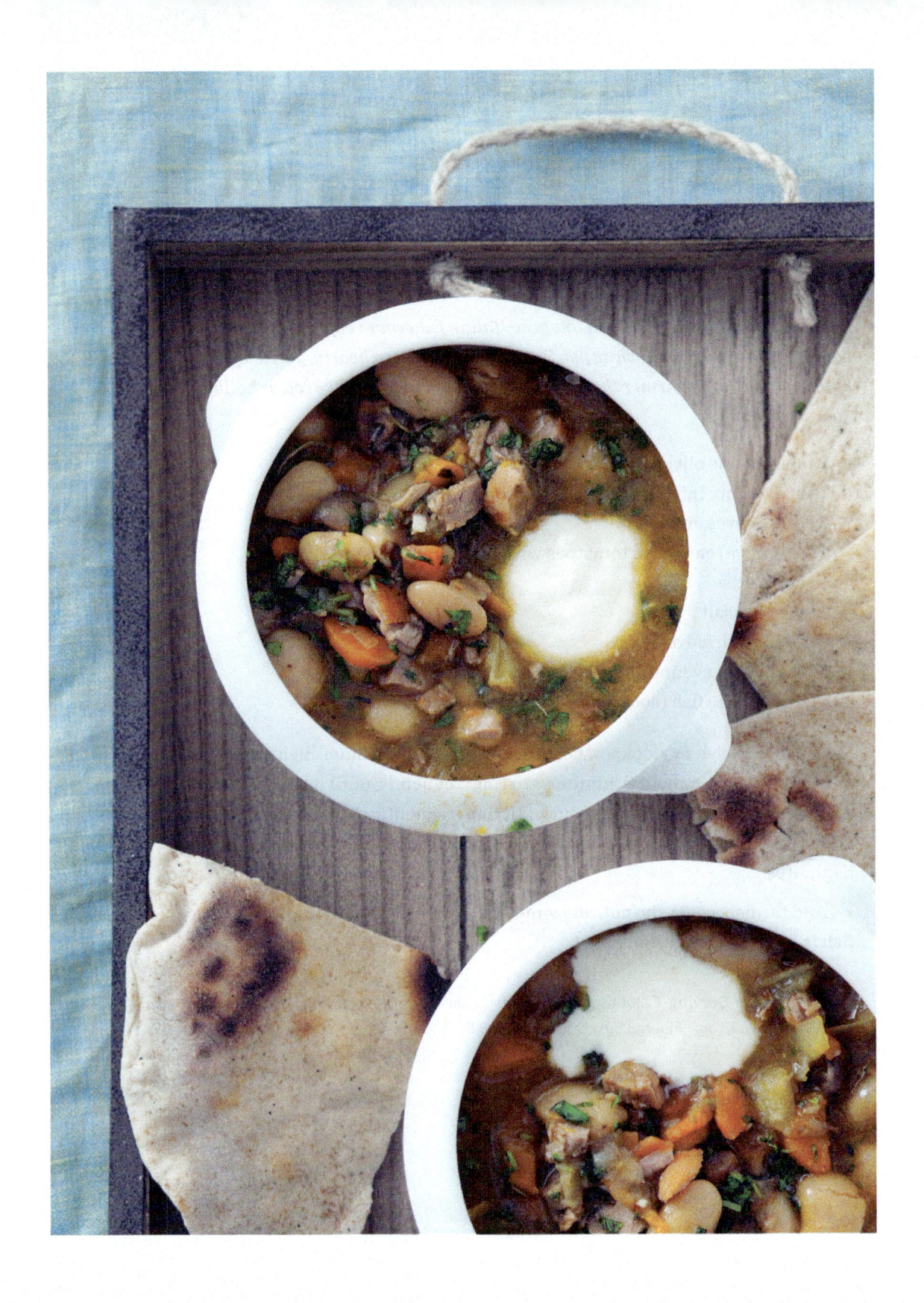

9

Meat and Poultry Dinners

Roasted Chicken and Vegetables   166
Chicken Enchiladas Verdes with Goat Cheese   168
Tandoori-Spiced Chicken Breast with Crisp Cucumber Salad   170
Roasted Chicken Breasts with Mustard and Greens   172
Thai-Style Curried Chicken Burgers   174
Chicken and White Bean Chili   175
Turkey Meatballs with Whole-Wheat Spaghetti and Spicy Tomato Sauce   177
Lamb Loin Chops with Yogurt-Mint Sauce   179
Goat Cheese and Spinach–Stuffed Pork Chops   181
Grilled Pineapple and Pork Skewers   183
Korean Stir-Fried Pork with Brown Rice   184
Pork Fried Brown Rice with Pineapple and Cashews   186
Bacon-Wrapped Meatloaf   188
Sesame-Soy Marinated Flank Steak with Wasabi-Spiked Cauliflower Purée   190
Quinoa Fried "Rice" with Flank Steak and Peas   192

Roasted Chicken and Vegetables

GLUTEN-FREE   DAIRY-FREE

Prep time: 15 minutes   **Cooking time:** 1 hour (plus 10 minutes to rest)

A perfectly roasted chicken is a beautiful thing: impressive enough for a special Sunday night dinner, a cinch to prepare, and a fantastic source of leftovers for future meals. This recipe includes succulent carrots and potatoes that are roasted right alongside the chicken, soaking up its flavorful juices and rounding out the meal. Get the biggest chicken you can at the butcher counter so you'll have enough meat left over for other dishes.

- 4 carrots, cut into 2-inch pieces
- 1 pound fingerling potatoes, halved
- ¼ cup olive oil, plus ¼ cup
- 4½ teaspoons salt, plus 1½ teaspoons
- 1 (4-pound) whole chicken
- 2 teaspoons freshly ground black pepper
- 2 garlic cloves, minced
- 1 lemon, quartered lengthwise

1. Preheat the oven to 475°F.

2. Put the carrots and potatoes in a roasting pan, drizzle with ¼ cup of olive oil, and sprinkle with 1½ teaspoons of the salt. Toss to coat.

3. Rinse the chicken inside and out and pat dry. Season it inside and out with the remaining 4½ teaspoons salt and the pepper.

4. In a small bowl, stir together the garlic and the remaining ¼ cup of olive oil. Rub the chicken all over with the oil mixture, inside and out. Put the lemon wedges inside the cavity of the chicken. Place the chicken, breast-side down,

on top of the vegetables in the roasting pan and roast for about 1 hour, until the chicken is golden brown and cooked through (a meat thermometer inserted into the thickest part of the thigh should register 175°F) and the vegetables are fork-tender.

5. Let the cooked chicken rest for 10 minutes. Remove it to a platter and carve as desired. Serve with the vegetables. Store any remaining chicken and vegetables separately in the refrigerator for up to 5 days.

Serves 8 / Per Serving Calories: 604   Total fat: 29.5g   Saturated fat: 6.5g   Protein: 67.2g   Carbohydrates: 15.1g   Fiber: 2.5g   Cholesterol: 202mg

COOKING TIP

To give your roast chicken a crisp skin and great flavor, and to ensure that it stays moist during cooking, dry-brine it a day ahead of time. Simply pat the chicken dry, cover it with about 2 tablespoons of salt, and refrigerate for 12 to 24 hours. Rinse off the salt and pat the chicken dry before roasting.

Chicken Enchiladas Verdes with Goat Cheese

GLUTEN-FREE

Prep time: 15 minutes   **Cooking time:** 25 minutes

A tangy and creamy green sauce made of tomatillos, jalapeño peppers, cilantro, and lime blankets chicken-filled soft corn tortillas for a spicy and comforting weeknight dinner. For a quick and satisfying meal, use leftover chicken from another meal. The Salsa Verde can also be prepared ahead, making this dish a cinch to put together quickly.

- 1 cup Salsa Verde (page 217), plus 1 cup, plus 3 tablespoons
- 2 cups shredded cooked chicken (from Roasted Chicken, page 164)
- ½ cup sour cream
- ½ cup crumbled goat cheese, plus ½ cup
- 2 tablespoons chopped fresh cilantro, plus 2 tablespoons
- 8 corn tortillas

1. Preheat the oven to 350°F. Spoon 3 tablespoons of the Salsa Verde sauce into a 9-inch square baking dish and spread it around with the back of a spoon.

2. In a large bowl, combine the chicken, 1 cup of the Salsa Verde, sour cream, ½ cup of the goat cheese, and 2 tablespoons of the cilantro. Set the remaining 1 cup Salsa Verde aside to pour over the top of the enchiladas.

3. Directly on a gas burner or in a clean, dry skillet over high heat, warm the tortillas one at a time. Put about 3 tablespoons of the chicken mixture in the center of one of the tortillas and roll it up into a cylinder. Transfer the roll to the baking pan and place it seam-side down in the dish. Repeat with the remaining tortillas and chicken. Cover the rolled-up enchiladas with the reserved Salsa Verde and the remaining ½ cup of goat cheese.

4. Bake for about 20 to 25 minutes, until the sauce is hot and bubbly and the cheese is melted and beginning to brown. Serve immediately, sprinkled with the remaining 2 tablespoons cilantro.

Serves 4 / Per Serving Calories: 497   Total fat: 24.6g   Saturated fat: 0.5g   Protein: 2.1g   Carbohydrates: 12.2g   Fiber: 7g   Cholesterol: 96mg

Tandoori-Spiced Chicken Breast with Crisp Cucumber Salad

GLUTEN-FREE

Prep time: 15 minutes (plus 2 to 24 hours to marinate the chicken)   **Cooking time:** 30 minutes

While chicken breast is lean and healthful, when cooked it can also be dry and bland. In this flavorful Indian dish, yogurt in the marinade tenderizes the chicken. A crisp cucumber salad is a refreshing accompaniment. This recipe makes enough chicken so that you'll have leftovers for two lunches later in the week.

- 3 cups plain yogurt
- 2 tablespoons peeled grated fresh ginger
- 2 tablespoon cooking oil, plus more for the pan
- 2 teaspoons ground cumin
- 1 teaspoon cayenne pepper
- 3 garlic cloves, minced
- 3¼ pounds skinless, boneless chicken breast
- 1 teaspoon salt

For the Cucumber Salad
- 2 medium cucumbers, halved lengthwise, seeded, and thinly sliced
- 1½ tablespoons salt
- 1 tablespoon white wine vinegar, plus 1 teaspoon
- 1 teaspoon honey

1. In a large bowl or resealable plastic bag, combine the yogurt, ginger, cooking oil, cumin, cayenne pepper, and garlic. Add the chicken and toss to coat. Marinate in the refrigerator for 2 hours up to overnight.

2. Preheat the oven to 400°F. Lightly coat a roasting pan with cooking oil.

3. Remove the chicken from the marinade and discard the marinade. Season the chicken pieces on both sides with the salt, and place in a single layer in the prepared roasting pan. Bake for about 30 minutes, turning once, until browned and cooked through (a meat thermometer when inserted in the fleshy part should register 175°F).

4. Meanwhile, make the cucumber salad. In a colander, toss the cucumber with the salt and let sit for about 20 minutes to render its liquid. Press any excess liquid out of the cucumber and then rinse with cold water and pat dry.

5. In a medium bowl, whisk the vinegar and honey to combine. Add the cucumber and toss to coat.

6. Reserve about two-thirds of the cooked chicken for later meals. Let cool to room temperature; then wrap, and refrigerate until ready to use.

7. Serve hot, accompanied by the cucumber salad.

Serves 4 (with leftover chicken for 2 meals) **/ Per Serving** Calories: 242   Total fat: 6.4g   Saturated fat: 2.3g   Protein: 38.9g   Carbohydrates: 7.2g   Fiber: 1.1g   Cholesterol: 99mg

Roasted Chicken Breasts with Mustard and Greens

GLUTEN-FREE   DAIRY-FREE

Prep time: 5 minutes   **Cooking time:** 1 hour

The beauty of a roasted chicken is that with just a little bit of prep, you can stick it in the oven and forget about it until it's time to eat. Here a mix of thighs and breasts get a blanketing of zesty Dijon mustard and a sprinkle of smoky paprika before being slipped into the hot oven. Just before the chicken is done, give the garlic-spiked greens a quick sauté, and voilà! Dinner is ready.

- 4 bone-in chicken breast halves
- 4 bone-in chicken thighs
- ½ cup Dijon mustard
- 2 teaspoons smoked paprika
- ¾ teaspoon salt
- ½ teaspoon freshly ground black pepper
- 2 tablespoons olive oil
- 1 pound Swiss chard, tough center ribs removed, leaves julienned
- 4 garlic cloves, minced

1. Preheat the oven to 375°F.

2. In a large baking dish, arrange the chicken pieces in a single layer and spread the mustard evenly over the chicken. Sprinkle the chicken with the paprika, salt, and pepper.

3. Bake the chicken for 45 to 55 minutes, until it is cooked through (a meat thermometer inserted into the fleshy part should register 175°F).

4. Meanwhile, in a large saucepan, heat the olive oil over medium-high heat. Add the Swiss chard and the garlic, cover, and cook until the greens are mostly wilted, about 2 minutes. Continue cooking the chard, stirring frequently, until completely wilted.

5. Transfer 2 or 3 of the chicken breasts (about ¾ pound of meat) to a storage container for another use. Serve the remaining chicken immediately on top of the greens.

Serves 4 (with leftover chicken for another use) **/ Per Serving** Calories: 327   Total fat: 17.1g   Saturated fat: 3.4g   Protein: 36.4g   Carbohydrates: 7.8g   Fiber: 3.4g   Cholesterol: 101mg

INGREDIENT TIP

Swiss chard is widely available and comes in a variety of colors, but you can substitute other hearty greens, such as kale, for the chard in this recipe. Mustard greens would add an additional dose of mustard flavor.

Thai-Style Curried Chicken Burgers

GLUTEN-FREE   DAIRY-FREE

Prep time: 10 minutes   **Cooking time:** 12 minutes

Ground chicken lets the flavors of garlic, ginger, and Thai curry paste shine in these quick, spicy burgers. If you don't have Thai curry paste, you could make your own paste using 2 tablespoons curry powder mixed with 1 tablespoon of olive oil.

- 1¼ pounds ground chicken
- 2 tablespoons chopped fresh cilantro
- 1 tablespoon peeled minced fresh ginger
- 2 garlic cloves, minced
- ½ red or yellow bell pepper, seeded, deribbed, and diced finely
- 1 to 2 tablespoons Thai red curry paste
- 1 teaspoon salt
- 2 teaspoons olive oil
- 2 medium tomatoes, sliced thinly
- ¼ cup Homemade Mayonnaise (page 217)
- 4 large lettuce leaves, such as butter or Bibb

1. In a medium bowl, add the chicken, cilantro, ginger, garlic, bell pepper, curry paste, and salt and mix well. Form the mixture into four patties. Brush the patties with the olive oil.

2. In a grill, grill pan, or skillet over medium-high heat, cook the burgers for about 6 minutes per side, until cooked through (a meat thermometer inserted into the center should read 175°F).

3. Serve the burgers with the tomatoes and Homemade Mayonnaise and wrapped in the lettuce leaves.

Serves 4 / Per Serving Calories: 494   Total fat: 19.1g   Saturated fat: 4.3g   Protein: 42.2g   Carbohydrates: 8.5g   Fiber: 1.1g   Cholesterol: 130mg

Chicken and White Bean Chili

GLUTEN-FREE   DAIRY-FREE

Prep time: 10 minutes   **Cooking time:** 40 minutes

Of the endless chili variations, this one stands out from the crowd. Made with chicken breast and green chiles and thickened with white beans, it's lighter than the traditional meat-heavy variety. If you like your chili spicier, add diced fresh jalapeño peppers along with the chopped green chiles. Top the chili with your favorite fixin's: sour cream or plain yogurt, shredded cheese, Cashew Cheese (page 224), Guacamole (page 212), chopped onion, sliced scallions, or chopped fresh cilantro would all be delicious additions.

- 1 tablespoon coconut oil
- 1 medium onion, chopped
- 1 pound boneless skinless chicken breasts, cut into bite-size pieces
- 2 garlic cloves, minced
- 2 medium carrots, diced
- 1 (4-ounce) can chopped green chiles
- 2 teaspoons ground cumin
- 2 teaspoons dried oregano
- 1½ teaspoons cayenne pepper
- 2 (14-ounce) cans chicken broth
- 2 (15-ounce) cans cannellini beans, rinsed and drained

1. In a Dutch oven or stockpot, heat the coconut oil over medium-high heat. Add the onion and cook for about 3 minutes, stirring frequently, until it begins to soften. Add the chicken and garlic and cook for about 4 minutes more, stirring and turning frequentlly, until the chicken is browned. Stir in the chiles, cumin, oregano, and cayenne pepper. Add the chicken broth and bring to a boil. Reduce the heat to low and let simmer. ➤

Meat and Poultry Dinners

Chicken and White Bean Chili, continued

2. Meanwhile, place about one-half of the beans in a medium bowl and, using a potato masher or a fork, mash the beans to a paste. Add the mashed beans to the pan along with the remaining one-half of the beans. Simmer for 20 to 30 minutes, uncovered, until the chicken is cooked through.

3. Serve hot with any desired toppings. Store leftovers in the refrigerator in an airtight container for up to 3 days or in the freezer for up to 3 months.

Serves 12 / Per Serving Calories: 448   Total fat: 7.2g   Saturated fat: 1.6g   Protein: 35.8g   Carbohydrates: 63.5g   Fiber: 25.9g   Cholesterol: 63.5mg

Turkey Meatballs with Whole-Wheat Spaghetti and Spicy Tomato Sauce

DAIRY-FREE

Prep time: 15 minutes   **Cooking time:** 20 minutes

Using ground turkey, toothsome whole-wheat pasta, and homemade Spicy Tomato Sauce turns this meal into a winner. The addition of Fresh Basil Pesto to the meatballs gives them a surprising burst of herby flavor. Lighter and far more nutritious than conventional spaghetti and meatballs, this hearty dish is undeniably delicious.

¾ pound ground turkey
2 tablespoons Fresh Basil Pesto (page 219; see Ingredient Tip, page 124)
½ teaspoon salt
½ teaspoon freshly ground black pepper
2 tablespoons olive oil, plus more for the parchment paper
2 cups Spicy Tomato Sauce (page 221)
8 ounces whole-wheat spaghetti

1. Preheat the oven to 375°F. Coat a piece of parchment paper with olive oil and line a large baking sheet with it.

2. In a medium bowl, combine the turkey, Fresh Basil Pesto, salt, and pepper and mix well. Wet your hands and form the mixture into 1½-inch balls. As you form the balls, place them on the prepared baking sheet with a bit of space between them. Brush the olive oil lightly over the tops of the meatballs.

3. Bake the meatballs for about 15 minutes, until they are lightly browned on the outside and cooked through (a meat thermometer inserted into the center of one meatball should register 175°F).

4. Meanwhile, in a large skillet, heat the Spicy Tomato Sauce over medium heat until hot. Reduce the heat to medium-low and let simmer slowly. ▸

Turkey Meatballs with Whole-Wheat Spaghetti and Spicy Tomato Sauce, continued

5. Fill a large pot about three-quarters full of water, and bring the water to a boil over high heat. Then cook the spaghetti according to the directions on the package.

6. Add the meatballs to the simmering sauce. Divide the cooked pasta evenly among four plates and top with ½ cup of the sauce and several meatballs. Serve immediately. Any leftovers can be stored, covered, in the refrigerator for up to 5 days.

Serves 4 / Per Serving Calories: 479 Total fat: 20.8g Saturated fat: 3.2g Protein: 34.6g Carbohydrates: 47g Fiber: 8g Cholesterol: 89mg

Lamb Loin Chops with Yogurt-Mint Sauce

GLUTEN-FREE

Prep time: 10 minutes **Cooking time:** 25 minutes

Spring is the traditional season for lamb, but it's delicious any season. It's at its most flavorful, moist, and tender when it is seared quickly in a hot pan and then cooked to medium-rare, as it is here. A tangy sauce of Greek yogurt and fresh mint is just the thing to temper the richness of the meat. A crisp green salad dressed with a piquant vinaigrette is all you need to round out this meal.

- 4 (2-inch-thick) lamb loin chops (or 8 [1-inch-thick] loin lamb chops), about 1½ pounds total
- 1 garlic clove, cut in half
- 1 teaspoon salt, plus ¾ teaspoon
- ½ teaspoon freshly ground black pepper, plus ½ teaspoon
- 1 tablespoon olive oil, plus 2 teaspoons
- ½ cup chopped fresh mint leaves
- 1 tablespoon freshly squeezed lemon juice
- 7 ounces plain Greek yogurt

1. Preheat the oven to 400°F.

2. Rub the lamb chops all over with the cut side of ½ garlic clove. Season the chops on both sides with ¾ teaspoon salt and ½ teaspoon pepper.

3. Coat an oven-safe grill pan or a large, heavy skillet with the 2 teaspoons of olive oil and heat over medium-high heat. When the pan is very hot, add the lamb and cook for 1 to 2 minutes per side, just until browned.

4. Place the pan in the oven and roast the lamb for 20 to 25 minutes, until it is cooked to the desired doneness (medium-rare is recommended; for well done, a meat thermometer inserted into the center of a chop should register 155°F). Let the lamb rest for 5 minutes before serving. ▶

Lamb Loin Chops with Yogurt-Mint Sauce, continued

5. Meanwhile, make the yogurt-mint sauce. Chop the remaining ½ garlic clove and add it to a food processor (or blender). Add the mint, the remaining 1 tablespoon olive oil, and the lemon juice and process to a paste. Add the yogurt and the remaining 1 teaspoon salt and ½ teaspoon pepper and pulse until smooth. Serve immediately, or cover and refrigerate for up to 3 days.

6. Serve the lamb chops hot, with a dollop of the yogurt-mint sauce.

Serves 4 / Per Serving Calories: 327   Total fat: 18.5g   Saturated fat: 6g   Protein: 34.3g   Carbohydrates: 4.9g   Fiber: 1g   Cholesterol: 113mg

Goat Cheese and Spinach–Stuffed Pork Chops

GLUTEN-FREE

Prep time: 10 minutes   **Cooking time:** 15 minutes

Stuffed with a mixture of spinach, tangy feta cheese, and sun-dried tomatoes, these juicy broiled pork chops are bursting with flavor. If you don't have a broiler, these pork chops would also be perfect cooked on an outdoor grill or grill pan. Be extra careful when you flip the chops so you keep the good stuffing in place.

- 2 teaspoons cooking oil
- 2 garlic cloves, minced, plus 2 garlic cloves, minced
- ¼ teaspoon salt, plus ½ teaspoon
- ¼ teaspoon freshly ground black pepper, plus ⅛ teaspoon
- 5 sun-dried oil-packed tomatoes, drained, patted dry, and diced
- 1 (10-ounce) package frozen chopped spinach, thawed and squeezed dry
- ½ cup (2 ounces) crumbled feta cheese
- ½ teaspoon grated fresh lemon zest
- 4 (4-ounce) boneless loin center-cut pork chops, trimmed
- 2 tablespoons freshly squeezed lemon juice
- 2 teaspoons Dijon mustard
- ¼ teaspoon dried oregano

1. Preheat the broiler.

2. In a large skillet over medium-high heat, heat the cooking oil. Add 2 of the minced garlic cloves and cook, stirring constantly, for about 1 minute. Add ¼ teaspoon of the salt, ⅛ teaspoon of the pepper, the sun-dried tomatoes, and the spinach and cook, stirring frequently, until the liquid has evaporated. Remove from the heat and stir in the feta cheese and lemon zest.

3. With a sharp knife, make a horizontal pocket in the middle of each pork chop. Fill each pocket with one-fourth of the spinach mixture. Season the outside of the pork chops with the remaining ½ teaspoon salt and ¼ teaspoon pepper. ▸

Goat Cheese and Spinach–Stuffed Pork Chops, continued

4. Put the chops on a broiler pan or roasting pan. In a small bowl, stir together the remaining 2 cloves of minced garlic, the lemon juice, mustard, and oregano and spread half of the mixture over the top of the chops. Broil for 6 minutes. Flip the chops over and brush the tops with the remaining mustard mixture. Cook under the broiler for 2 to 3 minutes more until cooked through. Let the chops rest for about 5 minutes before serving. Serve hot.

Serves 4 / Per Serving Calories: 386   Total fat: 21.4g   Saturated fat: 8.6g   Protein: 38g   Carbohydrates: 10.8g   Fiber: 3.7g   Cholesterol: 102mg

INGREDIENT TIP

Using frozen spinach saves time without sacrificing nutrition. If you prefer fresh spinach, you'll need about 1 pound of raw spinach before trimming off the stems (or about 12 ounces trimmed raw spinach) to equal 10 ounces of frozen spinach. To prepare raw spinach for use in this recipe, rinse it but don't dry it, and add it to the hot skillet along with the salt, pepper, and sun-dried tomatoes, and cook until the spinach is completely wilted and any water has evaporated.

Grilled Pineapple and Pork Skewers

DAIRY-FREE

Prep time: 15 minutes (plus 30 minutes to 24 hours to marinate)   **Cooking time:** 25 minutes

Pork and pineapple are a winning combination. The acid in the pineapple helps tenderize and flavor the pork, resulting in succulent chunks of meat and caramelized fruit that give you leftovers for another meal, such as Pork Fried Brown Rice with Pineapple and Cashews (page 186).

- 3 tablespoons low-sodium soy sauce
- 1 tablespoon peeled minced fresh ginger
- 1 garlic clove, minced
- ½ teaspoon freshly ground black pepper
- 1½ pounds boneless pork loin, cut into 1½-inch chunks
- 1 (15-ounce) can of unsweetened pineapple chunks packed in their own juice, drained (or 2 cups fresh pineapple chunks)

1. In a large bowl or resealable plastic bag, combine the soy sauce, ginger, garlic, and pepper. Add the pork and pineapple chunks and turn to coat well. Refrigerate for at least 30 minutes or as long as overnight.

2. Heat a grill or grill pan to high heat. Thread the pork and pineapple chunks onto metal skewers. Cook for about 10 minutes per side, until the pork and pineapple are browned and the pork is cooked through (a meat thermometer inserted into the side of one pork chunk should register 160°F).

3. Set one-third of the pork and pineapple aside for a later use. Cover and refrigerate for up to 3 days for another use.

4. Serve the skewers immediately. Leftovers can be stored in the refrigerator, covered, for up to 3 days.

Serves 4 / Per Serving (plus leftovers) Calories: 302   Total fat: 6.2g   Saturated fat: 2.1g   Protein: 46.2g   Carbohydrates: 14.9g   Fiber: 2.2g   Cholesterol: 124mg

Korean Stir-Fried Pork with Brown Rice

DAIRY-FREE

Prep time: 10 minutes (plus 1 hour to overnight to marinate the meat)   **Cooking time:** 1 hour

Inspired by the Korean dish called bulgogi, *this recipe uses lean pork in place of the traditional beef. The meat is marinated in soy sauce spiked with garlic and ginger. It gets a bit of spice from cayenne pepper and some sweetness from honey. For authentic Korean flavor, you could pass a bottle of the Korean fermented chili paste called* gochujang *at the table. If you can't find gochujang, use Sriracha sauce for added spice if you like.*

- ⅓ cup low-sodium soy sauce
- 2 tablespoons honey
- 1 tablespoon white wine vinegar
- 1 tablespoon sesame oil
- 1 teaspoon peeled minced fresh ginger
- ¼ to ½ teaspoon cayenne pepper
- 3 garlic cloves
- 2 pounds boneless pork loin, cut into thin strips
- 1 tablespoon coconut oil
- 1 small onion, thinly sliced
- 2 red or yellow bell peppers, seeded, deribbed, and cut into strips
- 2 cups hot cooked brown rice

1. In a large bowl or a resealable plastic bag, combine the soy sauce, honey, vinegar, sesame oil, ginger, cayenne pepper, and garlic cloves. Add the pork, turn to coat, and refrigerate for at least 1 hour or preferably overnight.

2. In a large skillet, heat the coconut oil over medium-high heat. Add the onion and cook for about 3 minutes, stirring frequently, until it begins to soften. Add the bell peppers and cook for 3 minutes, until they've begun to soften.

3. Drain the meat from the marinade (discard the marinade) and add to the pan. Cook for about 8 to 10 minutes, stirring frequently, until the meat is cooked through. Transfer one-half of the meat to a storage container and refrigerate for up to 3 days for a later use. Serve the meat and vegetables immediately over hot cooked brown rice.

Serves 4 (with leftover meat for a later use) / **Per Serving** Calories: 467 Total fat: 12.3g Saturated fat: 2.6g Protein: 35.5g Carbohydrates: 52.5g Fiber: 3.4g Cholesterol: 83mg

COOKING TIP

To cut meat into thin strips, use a very sharp knife and slice against the grain. To make meat easier to slice, pop it in the freezer for about 30 minutes before slicing.

Pork Fried Brown Rice with Pineapple and Cashews

DAIRY-FREE

Prep time: 5 minutes **Cooking time:** 15 minutes

Fried rice is quintessential comfort food—flavorful rice studded with savory morsels of meats and veggies. It's also a home cook's dream, one of those dishes that takes the leftovers hanging around in your refrigerator and brings them together in one delicious meal. This Thai-style fried rice includes bits of pineapple and cashews.

- 1 tablespoon coconut oil
- ½ small onion, diced
- 2 eggs, lightly beaten
- 2 cups cooked brown rice, cold
- 1 teaspoon sesame oil
- 1 tablespoon low-sodium soy sauce
- 8 ounces pork loin, cut into bite-size pieces
- 1 cup diced pineapple
- ¼ cup cashew halves

1. In a large skillet over medium-high heat, heat the coconut oil. Add the onion and cook for about 5 minutes, stirring frequently, until the onion is softened. Add the eggs and cook for about 3 minutes, stirring constantly with a spatula, until set. Transfer the egg-onion mixture to a bowl.

2. Add the brown rice, sesame oil, and soy sauce to the skillet and cook, using a spatula to break up the rice clumps. Cook for about 3 minutes, stirring frequently, until heated through.

3. Add the pork, pineapple, and cashews and cook for 2 to 3 minutes more, stirring frequently, until hot. Serve immediately. Store leftovers covered in the refrigerator for up to 3 days.

Serves 6 / Per Serving Calories: 419   Total fat: 14.3g   Saturated fat: 5.4g   Protein: 18.3g   Carbohydrates: 54.7g   Fiber: 3g   Cholesterol: 85mg

DIET VARIATION

The soy sauce in this dish contains gluten. To make the dish gluten-free, substitute gluten-free soy sauce or a gluten-free aminos sauce such as Bragg's Aminos.

Bacon-Wrapped Meatloaf

GLUTEN-FREE DAIRY-FREE

Prep time: 15 minutes   **Cooking time:** 55 minutes

A home-style classic, meatloaf is comfort food at its best. This recipe combines beef and pork for wonderful flavor and texture. The meatloaf is then wrapped with bacon strips, which keep the meat moist while adding delicious, smoky flavor and a crisp outer crust. Serve the meatloaf alongside puréed cauliflower and steamed or roasted vegetables.

- 2 pounds ground beef
- 1 pound ground pork
- 2 eggs, lightly beaten
- 1 cup almond flour
- 1 (6-ounce) can tomato paste
- 1 onion, chopped
- 1 cup jarred roasted red bell peppers, drained and minced
- 1 teaspoon ground cumin
- 1 teaspoon dried oregano
- 1½ teaspoons salt
- ¾ teaspoon freshly ground black pepper
- 12 slices natural smoked bacon

1. Preheat the oven to 350°F.

2. In a large bowl, and using clean hands, mix together the beef, pork, eggs, almond flour, tomato paste, onion, red peppers, cumin, oregano, salt, and pepper just until combined. Do not overwork the mixture or the meatloaf will become dry.

3. Pour the mixture into a 9-by-13-by-2-inch baking pan. Form into a loaf about 1½ inches tall, leaving some room around the sides where the juices can accumulate.

4. Arrange the bacon strips over the top so that they cover as much of the loaf as possible.

5. Bake for about 60 minutes (until a meat thermometer inserted in the center registers 160°F). Heat the broiler to high and broil the meatloaf for 10 minutes, watching carefully so it doesn't burn, until the bacon is crisp and browned. Let rest for 5 to 10 minutes. Remove the meatloaf to a platter and cut into eight to ten 1-inch slices. Serve immediately. Store leftovers, tightly wrapped, in the refrigerator for up to 5 days or in the freezer for up to 3 months.

Serves about 8 / Per Serving Calories: 449   Total fat: 22.6g   Saturated fat: 6.5g   Protein: 52g   Carbohydrates: 8.1g   Fiber: 2.5g   Cholesterol: 172mg

INGREDIENT TIP

You can use fresh red bell peppers instead of jarred peppers if you wish. Choose 2 or 3 good-size ones, remove the seeds and ribs and cut them into thin slices, and then cook them, skin-side up, under the broiler until the skin is charred, about 5 minutes. Put them in a bowl, cover with plastic wrap, and let sit for 10 minutes to loosen the charred skin. Peel and discard the charred skin and proceed with the recipe as written.

Sesame-Soy Marinated Flank Steak with Wasabi-Spiked Cauliflower Purée

GLUTEN-FREE   DAIRY-FREE

Prep time: 15 minutes (plus overnight to marinate steak)   **Cooking time:** 22 minutes

Lean and flavorful, flank steak takes especially well to marinating and grilling. Better still, it's a budget-conscious cut that makes for tasty leftovers that can be used in salads, sandwiches, and other dishes. Here, flank steak is marinated in soy sauce and sesame oil with a touch of honey, ginger, and garlic and then grilled to medium-rare. The wasabi-spiked cauliflower purée is a light and flavorful satisfying side dish that's easier on the waistline than classic mashed potatoes. Marinate the steak the night before to infuse it with flavor. This recipe makes enough steak for two meals.

For the Steak

1½ pounds flank steak

Salt

Freshly ground black pepper

1 teaspoon thinly sliced peeled fresh ginger

1 garlic clove, thinly sliced

¼ cup low-sodium soy sauce

1 tablespoon sesame oil

1 teaspoon honey

For the Cauliflower

1 large head cauliflower, leaves and core removed and separated into florets

½ to 1 tablespoon wasabi powder mixed to a paste with an equal amount of water

1 tablespoon olive oil

1 teaspoon salt

½ teaspoon freshly ground black pepper

1. To marinate the steak, season it on both sides with salt and pepper. In a large bowl or resealable plastic bag, combine the ginger, garlic, soy sauce, sesame oil, and honey and mix well. Add the steak and turn to coat. Refrigerate overnight.

2. Preheat a grill or grill pan to medium-high heat.

3. Bring the steak to room temperature by setting it on the counter for about 20 minutes before grilling.

4. To make the cauliflower purée, fill a saucepan fitted with a steamer basket with about 2 inches of water and bring to a boil over medium-high heat. Put the cauliflower florets in the steamer basket, cover the pan, and cook for 8 to 10 minutes, just until the cauliflower is fork-tender. Transfer the cauliflower to a food processor (or blender, or put it in a large bowl and use an immersion blender) and add the wasabi paste, olive oil, salt, and pepper and blend to a smooth purée. Adjust the seasoning if needed.

5. To grill the flank steak, remove it from the marinade, letting the excess marinade run off, and place it on the grill or grill pan. Grill for 4 to 6 minutes per side, until cooked to medium-rare (cook 1 or 2 minutes longer on each side if you prefer a more well-done steak). Set aside on a cutting board and let rest for about 5 minutes. Slice off one-third of the steak and let it come to room temperature before wrapping and storing it in the refrigerator for another use. Cut the remaining steak against the grain into ¼-inch-thick slices and serve the cauliflower purée alongside.

Serves 4 (plus 8 ounces additional steak for another use) **/ Per Serving** Calories: 326 Total fat: 14.8g   Saturated fat: 4.7g   Protein: 36.1g   Carbohydrates: 12.9g   Fiber: 5.3g Cholesterol: 62mg

Quinoa Fried "Rice" with Flank Steak and Peas

GLUTEN-FREE DAIRY-FREE

Prep time: 10 minutes   **Cooking time:** 12 minutes

More flavorful and more nutritious than the usual steamed white rice, quinoa makes a satisfying substitute grain to use in the classic fried rice preparation. It's best to use leftover cooked quinoa for this dish since it should be cold when it is added to the pan. This recipe also utilizes leftover cooked flank steak.

2 teaspoons cooking oil
2 teaspoons sesame oil
¼ small onion, chopped
2 carrots, chopped
3 garlic cloves, minced
1 teaspoon peeled minced fresh ginger
3 cups cooked quinoa (see Cooking Tip, page 96)
3 tablespoons low-sodium soy sauce
2 eggs, lightly beaten
8 ounces Sesame-Soy Marinated Flank Steak (page 190)
½ cup frozen peas

1. In a large skillet, heat the cooking oil and sesame oil over medium-high heat. Add the onion and carrots and cook for about 2 minutes, stirring frequently, until they begin to soften. Add the garlic and ginger and cook for 2 minutes.

2. Stir in the cooked quinoa and cook for 2 minutes, stirring frequently, to heat through. Add the soy sauce and stir to mix. Push the quinoa mixture to the side of the pan, and add the eggs to the empty side of the pan. Cook for about 2 minutes, stirring with a spatula, until just cooked through; then toss with the quinoa-vegetable mixture.

3. Add the flank steak and peas, and cook another 3 minutes or so until heated through. Serve hot. Store any leftovers, covered, in the refrigerator for up to 3 days.

Serves 4 / Per Serving Calories: 545   Total fat: 19.9g   Saturated fat: 4.4g   Protein: 32.1g   Carbohydrates: 59.6g   Fiber: 7.6g   Cholesterol: 113mg

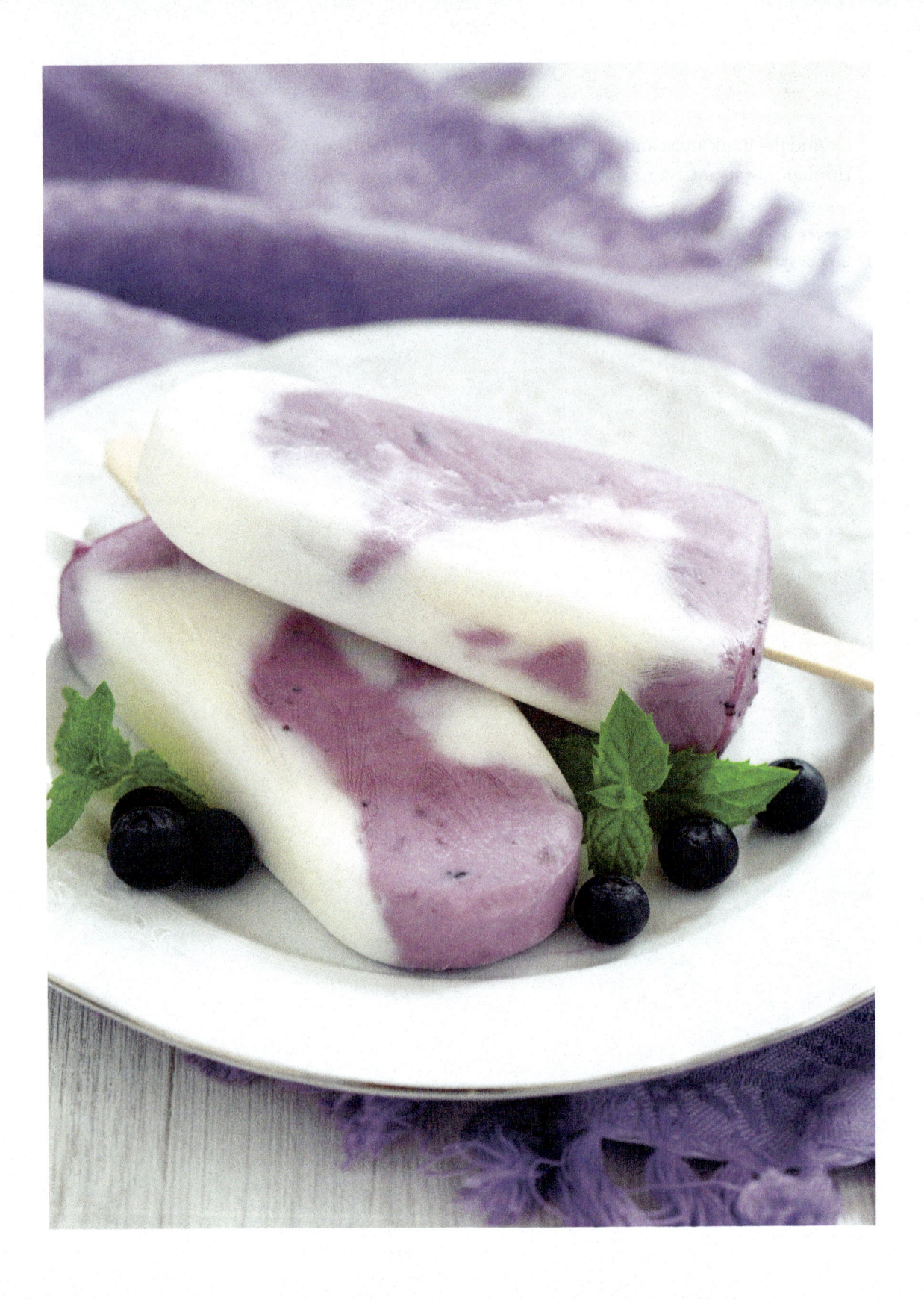

10

Dessert

Yogurt Blueberry Ice Pops   196
Banana Maple Nut "Ice Cream"   197
Cocoa Almond Pudding   198
Peanut Butter Oatmeal Cookies   199
Apple Crisp with Fresh Ginger   200
Berry Crumb Cake   202
Banana Chocolate Tart   204
Molten Chocolate Cakes   206
Rich Chocolate Fudge   207
Mini Cheesecakes in Caramel Sauce   208

Yogurt Blueberry Ice Pops

VEGETARIAN   GLUTEN-FREE

Prep time: 5 minutes (plus at least 4 hours to freeze)   **Cooking time:** None

Made of yogurt, fruit, and honey, all frozen into an easy-to-eat, hand-held ice pop, this is one healthful treat that everyone in the family is sure to love. Blueberries give this version a beautiful purple hue, but you could use just about any fruit you like. Blackberries or strawberries would be just as pretty, but peaches or nectarines would be delicious as well. Use ice pop molds if you have them, or small cups with sticks.

- 2 cups plain yogurt or Greek yogurt
- ¼ cup honey
- 1 teaspoon vanilla extract (optional)
- 1 cup frozen blueberries

1. In a blender, combine the yogurt, honey, and vanilla (if using) and blend. Transfer half of the mixture to a pitcher or large measuring cup with a spout. Add the blueberries to the yogurt mixture remaining in the pitcher and blend to a smooth purée.

2. Pour a bit of the plain yogurt mixture into six ice pop molds, or small cups. Top with some of the blueberry-yogurt mixture. Repeat, layering plain yogurt and blueberry yogurt in uneven amounts until all of the molds are filed. Insert the lid of the ice pop mold or sticks and freeze for at least 4 hours. These can be stored in the freezer for up to 3 months.

Makes 6 ice pops / Per Serving Calories: 117   Total fat: 1.1g   Saturated fat: 0.8g   Protein: 4.9g   Carbohydrates: 21g   Fiber: 0.6g   Cholesterol: 5mg

Banana Maple Nut "Ice Cream"

VEGETARIAN   VEGAN   GLUTEN-FREE   DAIRY-FREE

Prep time: 10 minutes (plus 2 hours to freeze)   **Cooking time:** None

How many times have you tossed a bunch of overripe bananas because you didn't have the time or inclination to whip up a batch of banana bread? Next time, peel the bananas, break them into chunks, and stick them in a resealable, freezer-safe bag in the freezer. On the next hot day, you'll be able to whip up this sweet, refreshing, and healthful dessert. Made with just four nutritious, all-natural ingredients, it will satisfy your ice cream cravings and then some.

- 4 ripe bananas, peeled, broken into chunks, and frozen
- 3 tablespoons maple syrup
- 1 teaspoon vanilla extract
- 1/3 cup walnut pieces

1. In the bowl of a food processor (or blender), add the bananas, maple syrup, and vanilla, and process until smooth and creamy, scraping down the sides of the bowl as needed. Transfer the mixture to a bowl and stir in the walnuts.

2. Pour into a freezer-safe container and freeze for at least 2 hours, stirring every once in a while.

3. Serve frozen. The dessert can be kept in the freezer for up to 3 months.

Serves 4 / Per Serving Calories: 212   Total fat: 6.2g   Saturated fat: 0g   Protein: 3.7g   Carbohydrates: 38.1g   Fiber: 4.2g   Cholesterol: 0mg

Cocoa Almond Pudding

VEGETARIAN   GLUTEN-FREE   DAIRY-FREE

Prep time: 2 minutes   **Cooking time:** 10 minutes

Full of chocolaty flavor, this creamy, rich pudding is made without dairy or eggs (or gluten, for that matter!). It gets its custardy texture from arrowroot starch and is sweetened with honey. For a vegan variation, use maple syrup or agave syrup instead of honey.

- 2 cups unsweetened almond milk
- ¼ cup honey
- ½ cup unsweetened cocoa powder
- 3 tablespoons arrowroot starch
- 1 teaspoon vanilla extract

1. In a medium saucepan over medium heat, add the almond milk and honey and whisk to combine; then slowly whisk in the cocoa powder and arrowroot. Bring to a boil and cook for about 8 minutes, stirring constantly, until the mixture thickens.

2. Remove from the heat and stir in the vanilla. Cool to room temperature and pour into four dessert bowls. Serve immediately, or refrigerate, covered, for several hours and serve chilled.

Serves 4 / Per Serving Calories: 128   Total fat: 2.7g   Saturated fat: 0.9g   Protein: 2.7g   Carbohydrates: 29.2g   Fiber: 4.3g   Cholesterol: 0mg

Peanut Butter Oatmeal Cookies

VEGETARIAN GLUTEN-FREE DAIRY-FREE

Prep time: 10 minutes (plus 30 minutes to chill dough)   **Cooking time:** 12 minutes

These easy-to-make cookies hit the spot when you crave a sweet nibble. Keep them around for after-school treats for the kids or a simple after-dinner dessert. You can use either creamy or chunky peanut butter, just make sure it's all-natural with no sugar, palm oil, or other additives.

- ⅔ cup old-fashioned rolled oats
- ½ teaspoon ground cinnamon
- 1 teaspoon baking soda
- 1 egg, lightly beaten
- 1 cup all-natural peanut butter, at room temperature
- ½ cup coconut sugar

1. In a medium bowl, add the oats, cinnamon, and baking soda and stir to combine. In another medium bowl, add the egg, peanut butter, and coconut sugar and mix with a wooden spoon until well combined. Add the oats mixture to the peanut butter mixture and stir to combine. Chill the dough mixture in the refrigerator for 30 minutes.

2. Preheat the oven to 350°F. Line two large baking sheets with parchment paper.

3. Drop the dough by heaping tablespoons onto the prepared baking sheets, leaving about 3 inches between the cookies. With the back of a spoon, press the dough balls to flatten slightly.

4. Bake for 10 to 12 minutes, until the cookies begin to look crisp. Let the cookies cool on the baking sheet for about 10 minutes; then transfer them to a wire rack to cool completely. Serve immediately, or store in an airtight container at room temperature for up to 1 week.

Makes about 28 cookies / Per Serving Calories: 179   Total fat: 11.5g   Saturated fat: 2.4g   Protein: 6.4g   Carbohydrates: 15.4g   Fiber: 1.8g   Cholesterol: 14mg

Apple Crisp with Fresh Ginger

VEGETARIAN

Prep time: 15 minutes   **Cooking time:** 25 minutes

Sweet-tart apples combined with the kick of fresh ginger make this apple crisp stand out from the crowd. The topping, too, is unique in that it is made with yogurt instead of butter. A gel made of ground flaxseed and water gives the topping structure so that it crisps up nicely. This is one dessert you can eat totally guilt-free—you'll even get a serving of fresh fruit while you're at it. Serve with a dollop of Whipped Coconut Cream (page 226), if desired.

Cooking oil, for the baking dish
½ cup ground flaxseed
¼ cup water
4 medium apples, such as Granny Smith, thinly sliced
Juice of 1 freshly squeezed lemon
2 tablespoons peeled minced fresh ginger
2¼ cups old-fashioned rolled oats
2 tablespoons coconut sugar
2 tablespoons whole-wheat flour
⅓ cup plain yogurt or Greek yogurt

1. Preheat the oven to 400°F. Lightly oil an 8-inch square baking dish.

2. In a large bowl, combine the flaxseed and water and let sit until it forms a gel, about 5 minutes.

3. In a large bowl, toss the apples with the lemon juice and ginger. Spread the apple mixture in an even layer in the prepared baking dish.

4. To the bowl with the flaxseed mixture, add the oats, coconut sugar, and flour and stir to combine. Add the yogurt and stir until the topping mixture clumps together.

5. Dollop the topping over the apples in the baking dish.

6. Bake for 20 to 25 minutes, until the fruit is fork-tender and hot and bubbly and the topping begins to brown. Serve hot.

7. Store leftovers tightly covered in the refrigerator for up to 3 days. To serve, reheat, uncovered, in a 400°F oven for 10 to 15 minutes until hot.

Serves 8 / Per Serving Calories: 193   Total fat: 4g   Saturated fat: 0.8g   Protein: 6.1g   Carbohydrates: 32.9g   Fiber: 6.4g   Cholesterol: 1mg

Berry Crumb Cake

VEGETARIAN   GLUTEN-FREE   DAIRY-FREE

Prep time: 15 minutes   **Cooking time:** 60 minutes

This delicious crumb cake, made with juicy blueberries and a sweet crumb topping, works as a dessert or as a coffee cake. It's wonderful with fresh berries when they're in season, but frozen berries work perfectly. You could also substitute another fruit such as blackberries or diced peaches for the blueberries. Serve with a dollop of Whipped Coconut Cream (page 226), if desired.

For the Topping

½ cup coconut sugar
⅓ cup almond flour
¼ teaspoon ground cinnamon
Pinch of salt
2 tablespoons coconut oil

For the Cake

½ cup coconut oil, plus more for the pan
2 cups almond flour
1 cup coconut sugar
2 teaspoons baking powder
½ teaspoon salt
2 eggs
⅓ cup unsweetened almond milk
1 teaspoon vanilla extract
1 tablespoon apple cider vinegar
2 cups frozen blueberries (do not thaw)

1. Preheat the oven to 350°F. Coat an 8-inch square baking pan with coconut oil.

2. To make the crumb topping, in the bowl of a food processor (or blender), add the coconut sugar, almond flour, cinnamon, salt, and coconut oil and pulse until the mixture resembles a coarse meal.

3. To make the cake, in the bowl of a stand mixer (or in a large bowl using a hand mixer), add the coconut oil, almond flour, coconut sugar, baking powder, and salt and mix until crumbly.

4. Put the eggs, almond milk, vanilla, and vinegar in a medium bowl and whisk to combine. Add the egg mixture to the almond flour mixture and mix until just combined.

5. Pour the cake batter into the prepared pan. Sprinkle the blueberries evenly over the top, and then sprinkle the crumb topping over the berries.

6. Bake for 55 to 60 minutes, until a toothpick inserted into the center comes out clean. Remove from the oven and let cool completely in the pan before serving. Cut into squares to serve. Wrap the leftovers tightly in plastic wrap and store in the refrigerator for up to 3 days or freeze for up to 3 months. Thaw at room temperature before serving.

Serves 12 / Per Serving Calories: 274   Total fat: 17.6g   Saturated fat: 11.7g   Protein: 2.9g   Carbohydrates: 30.1g   Fiber: 1.6g   Cholesterol: 27mg

Banana Chocolate Tart

VEGETARIAN   GLUTEN-FREE   DAIRY-FREE

Prep time: 15 minutes (plus 1 hour 15 minutes for chilling)   **Cooking time:** 10 minutes

Made without dairy products, this rich dark chocolate tart has an almond flour crust that is gluten free. Its filling is enriched with silken tofu, which gives it a creamy mouthfeel (plus a protein boost). Sweetened with maple syrup, dates, and coconut sugar instead of refined sugar, this clean dessert will rival your old favorites.

For the Crust
1½ cups almond flour
¼ cup unsweetened cocoa powder
¼ cup maple syrup
¼ cup coconut oil
¼ teaspoon salt

For the Filling
½ cup pitted dates
⅔ cup silken tofu
6 tablespoons unsweetened cocoa powder
3 tablespoons honey
½ teaspoon vanilla extract
1 large banana, thinly sliced

1. To make the crust, in the bowl of a food processor (or blender), add the almond flour, cocoa powder, maple syrup, coconut oil, and salt and process for 1 minute until the mixture holds together when pinched. Press the mixture into an even layer in the bottom and up the sides of a 9-inch, removable-bottom tart pan. Chill in the refrigerator for 15 minutes.

2. While the crust is chilling, make the filling. In a small saucepan, put the dates and cover by 1 inch with cold water. Bring to a boil over medium-high heat; then reduce the heat to medium-low and simmer for about 10 minutes. Transfer the

dates and ¼ cup of the cooking water to the bowl of the food processor. Add the tofu, cocoa powder, honey, and vanilla and process until smooth. Transfer the filling to the chilled crust, smoothing with a rubber spatula, and chill for at least 1 hour.

3. Remove the ring around the bottom of the tart and place on a platter. Arrange the banana slices over the top just before serving. Serve chilled. Store in the refrigerator, wrapped in plastic wrap, for up to 5 days.

Serves 6 / Per Serving Calories: 268   Total fat: 14.3g   Saturated fat: 8.9g   Protein: 4.7g   Carbohydrates: 37.7g   Fiber: 5.6g   Cholesterol: 0mg

DIET VARIATION

To make this recipe vegan, replace the honey with an equal amount of coconut sugar, maple syrup, or other natural sweetener.

Molten Chocolate Cakes

VEGETARIAN   DAIRY-FREE

Prep time: 10 minutes   **Cooking time:** 10 minutes

These single-serving cakes are memorable enough to be special, but easy enough to make anytime. Use a pure dark cocoa for best results. Serve with a dollop of Whipped Coconut Cream (page 226), if desired.

- Coconut oil, for the ramekins
- ¼ cup unsweetened cocoa powder, plus 1 tablespoon
- ½ cup coconut sugar
- 2 tablespoons honey
- 1 teaspoon vanilla extract
- 2 tablespoons coconut oil, melted
- 1 egg
- 1 egg white
- ½ cup whole-wheat flour

1. Preheat the oven to 400°F. Lightly coat four 4-ounce ramekins or custard cups with coconut oil.

2. In a medium bowl, add the cocoa powder, coconut sugar, honey, vanilla, and melted coconut oil and whisk together.

3. In a small bowl, add the whole egg and egg white and whisk to beat lightly. Add the eggs to the cocoa mixture and whisk until smooth.

4. Stir the flour into the mixture just until completely incorporated, but be careful not to overmix. Spoon the batter into the prepared ramekins, dividing evenly, and put them on a baking sheet.

5. Bake for about 10 minutes, until the sides are firm and the center is set but still soft. Remove the cakes from the oven and invert each ramekin onto a serving plate. Let stand for 5 minutes before removing the ramekin. Serve warm.

Makes 4 mini cakes / Per Serving Calories: 419   Total fat: 13.2g   Saturated fat: 7g   Protein: 7g   Carbohydrates: 73.9g   Fiber: 3.3g   Cholesterol: 41mg

Rich Chocolate Fudge

VEGETARIAN   VEGAN   GLUTEN-FREE   DAIRY-FREE

Prep time: 5 minutes (plus 15 minutes to soak the dried fruit and 2 hours to chill)
Cooking time: None

Moist, sweet dates effectively stand in for sugar in this decadent fudge. You can use any type of date you like for this recipe, but Medjool dates, if they're available, are the best. Extra plump, with a crinkly skin, sticky, sweet flesh, and a flavor reminiscent of rich caramel, they provide all the sweetness you need with a rounder, richer flavor than refined sugar.

- ½ cup pitted dates
- ½ cup raisins
- ½ cup unsweetened almond milk
- 1 cup all-natural peanut butter (or almond butter)
- ½ cup unsweetened cocoa powder
- ½ cup unsweetened shredded coconut
- ¼ teaspoon vanilla extract

1. Line an 8-inch square baking pan with parchment paper.

2. In a medium bowl, put the dates and raisins and pour the almond milk over them. Let soak for 15 minutes.

3. Transfer the dates and raisins, along with the soaking liquid, to the bowl of a food processor (or blender) and process to a paste. Transfer the mixture back to the soaking bowl. Add the peanut butter, cocoa powder, coconut, and vanilla and stir to mix well.

4. Press the mixture into the prepared pan. Chill in the refrigerator for at least 2 hours. Cut into small squares to serve. Store leftovers wrapped tightly in the refrigerator for up to 2 weeks.

Serves 8 / Per Serving Calories: 313   Total fat: 22.3g   Saturated fat: 8.5g   Protein: 10.2g   Carbohydrates: 21g   Fiber: 5.7g   Cholesterol: 0mg

Mini Cheesecakes in Caramel Sauce

VEGETARIAN   GLUTEN-FREE

Prep time: 10 minutes (plus 30 minutes to cool)   **Cooking time:** 30 minutes

These creamy cheesecakes in caramel sauce are reminiscent of silky, sweet flan or crème caramel. The white custard and golden syrup look stunning on a plate, making these little gems impressive enough to serve at the fanciest of dinner parties. But made with just four all-natural ingredients and sweetened with coconut sugar, they're healthful enough to eat anytime you please.

- ⅓ cup coconut sugar, plus ⅓ cup
- 2 tablespoons water
- 6 ounces whipped cream cheese
- 2 eggs
- ¼ cup plain Greek yogurt

1. Preheat the oven to 350°F. Set six 4-ounce ramekins in a 9-by-13-by-2-inch baking pan.

2. In a small saucepan, combine ⅓ cup of the coconut sugar and the 2 tablespoons water and bring to a boil over medium-high heat. Boil for 45 to 60 seconds, stirring constantly until the sauce thickens slightly and becomes syrupy. Spoon the mixture into the ramekins, dividing equally.

3. In the bowl of a food processor (or blender), add the cream cheese, eggs, yogurt, and the remaining ⅓ cup coconut sugar and pulse until combined. Spoon the cream cheese mixture into the prepared ramekins on top of the sugar syrup, dividing equally. Carefully pour warm water into the pan to come halfway up the sides of the ramekins.

4. Bake for 25 to 30 minutes, until the cream cheese mixture is set and a knife inserted into the center comes out clean. Turn the oven off, but leave the cheesecakes in the oven until the oven cools to room temperature, about 30 minutes.

5. Run a knife around the outside edge of one of the cheesecakes to separate it from the ramekin. Place the ramekin in a shallow pan of very hot water to loosen the caramel, letting it sit for about 5 minutes. Carefully invert the cheesecake onto a serving plate. The loosened caramel will run out over the top of the cheesecake to make a sauce. Repeat for the remaining cheesecakes. Serve immediately.

6. To store extra cheesecakes, leave them in their ramekins, cover with plastic wrap, and refrigerate for up to 3 days. Bring to room temperature, loosen the cheesecakes from the sides of the ramekins, and set in a hot water bath for about 5 minutes before serving.

Makes 6 mini cheesecakes / Per Serving Calories: 149   Total fat: 2g   Saturated fat: 0.8g   Protein: 8g   Carbohydrates: 26g   Fiber: 0.6g   Cholesterol: 66mg

TIP TO DOUBLE OR HALVE THE RECIPE

If you're serving these cheesecakes for a party, simply double (or triple) the ingredients and follow the directions as written using twice (or three times) as many ramekins. You can also halve the recipe by cutting the ingredients in half and using three ramekins instead of six.

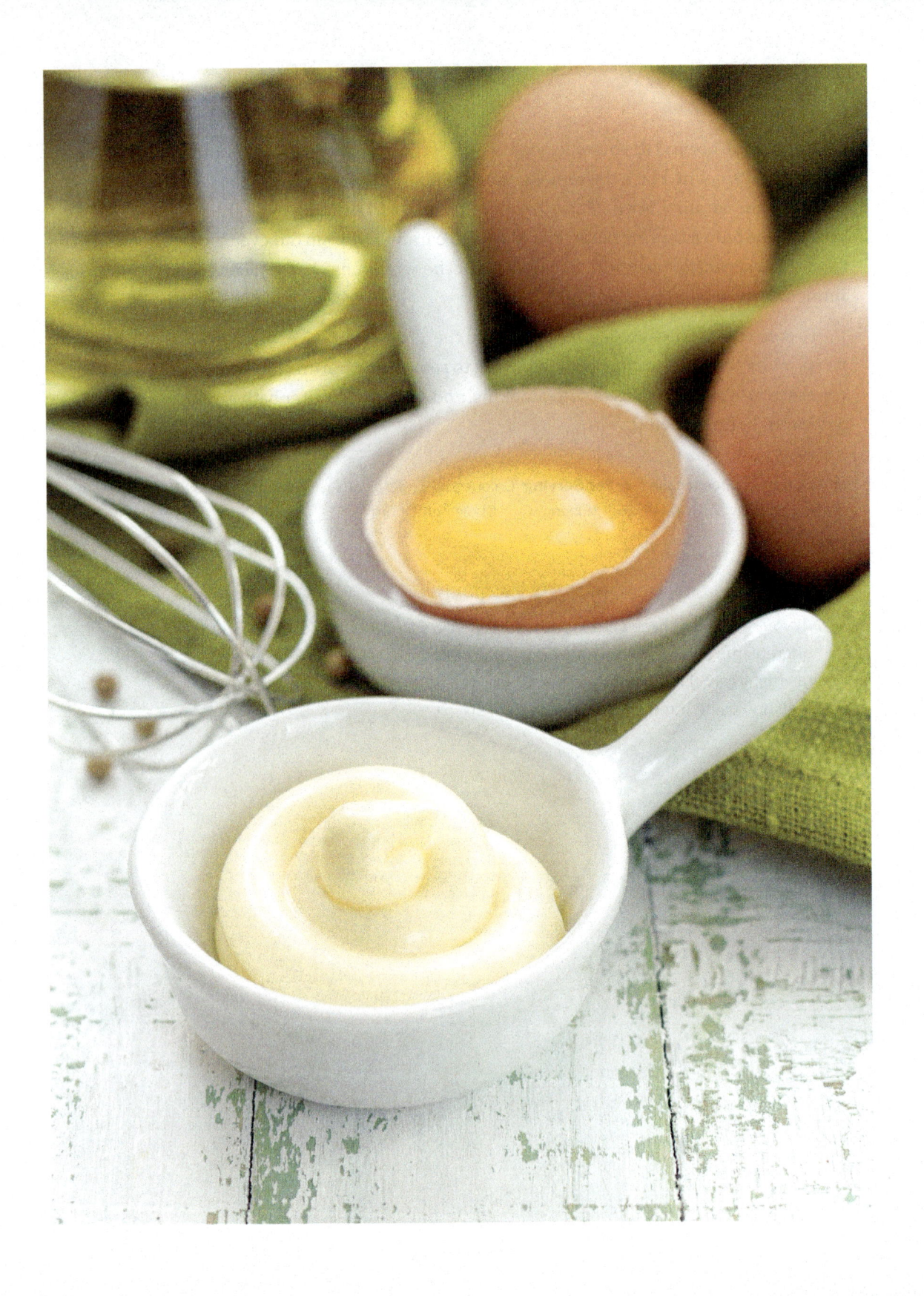

11

Kitchen Staples
Condiments, Sauces, and Dressings

Guacamole   212
Pico de Gallo   213
Balsamic Vinaigrette   214
Lemon Vinaigrette   215
Yogurt Dressing   216
Homemade Mayonnaise   217
Salsa Verde   218
Fresh Basil Pesto   219
Romesco Sauce   220
Spicy Tomato Sauce   221
Chicken Broth   222
Vegetable Broth   223
Cashew Cheese   224
Homemade Almond Milk   225
Whipped Coconut Cream   226

Guacamole

VEGETARIAN   VEGAN   GLUTEN-FREE   DAIRY-FREE

Prep time: 10 minutes   **Cooking time:** None

A perfectly ripe, creamy avocado needs very little to turn it into an addictive guacamole. This version uses only a splash of lime juice, diced tomato and onion, and some cayenne pepper to jazz it up. Use the guacamole as a dip for chips, as a sandwich spread, or to top tacos, burritos, or enchiladas.

- 4 ripe Haas avocados
- 1 medium tomato, seeded and finely diced
- ½ cup finely diced red onion
- 3 tablespoons freshly squeezed lime juice
- 1 teaspoon salt
- ½ teaspoon cayenne pepper

In a medium bowl, mash the avocado with a fork until mostly smooth. Stir in the tomato, onion, lime juice, salt, and cayenne pepper. Serve immediately. To store leftovers, cover the bowl with plastic wrap and press the wrap directly onto the guacamole, pressing out any air bubbles. Store in the refrigerator for up to 1 day.

Makes about 3 cups (about 8 servings) / **Per Serving** Calories: 210   Total fat: 19.6g   Saturated fat: 4.1g   Protein: 2g   Carbohydrates: 9.6g   Fiber 7g   Cholesterol: 0mg

INGREDIENT TIP

Be sure to use Haas avocados (the kind with bumpy black skin) as they have the perfect creamy texture for guacamole. Choose fruit that is firm but has a bit of give when you gently press the stem end with your thumb.

Pico de Gallo

VEGETARIAN   VEGAN   GLUTEN-FREE   DAIRY-FREE

Prep time: 10 minutes   **Cooking time:** None

An outstanding pico de gallo (also called salsa fresca, or fresh salsa) is fresh and bright, with a touch of heat and the herbaceous bite of cilantro. It's delicious as a dip for chips or on tacos or burritos, but it can also be used as a sauce for grilled fish or chicken, spooned over eggs, or used to spice up a bowl of rice and beans.

- ½ cup finely diced onion
- 1 garlic clove, minced
- Juice of 1 freshly squeezed lime
- ½ teaspoon salt
- 1 jalapeño pepper, seeded and diced
- 4 plum tomatoes, diced
- ½ cup chopped fresh cilantro

1. In a small bowl, put the onion, garlic, and lime juice and stir to combine. Stir in the salt and let rest for a few minutes to soften the onions and meld the flavors.

2. Stir in the jalapeño pepper, tomatoes, and cilantro. Taste and add more salt, if needed. Cover and refrigerator for 1 to 2 hours to let the flavors meld. Serve immediately, or store tightly covered in the refrigerator for up to 3 days.

Makes about 2½ cups (about 4 servings) / Per Serving Calories: 36   Total fat: 0.3g   Saturated fat: 0g   Protein: 1.7g   Carbohydrates: 7.9g   Fiber 1.7g   Cholesterol: 0mg

Balsamic Vinaigrette

VEGETARIAN   VEGAN   GLUTEN-FREE   DAIRY-FREE

Prep time: 3 minutes   **Cooking time:** None

Bottled salad dressings—even the so-called healthful ones—are generally loaded with sugar and other additives. This simple sweet-tart vinaigrette takes just a few minutes to whip up and uses only all-natural, unprocessed ingredients that you probably have in your pantry. Best of all, you can use it to dress just about any salad combination you can dream up.

- ¼ cup balsamic vinegar
- 3 tablespoons Dijon mustard
- 1½ teaspoons salt
- ¾ teaspoon freshly ground black pepper
- 6 tablespoons olive oil

In a small bowl, whisk together the vinegar, mustard, salt, and pepper. Add the olive oil and whisk until the dressing is emulsified. Vinaigrette can be stored in the refrigerator for up to 2 weeks. Bring to room temperature and shake or whisk well before using.

Makes about 1 cup (about eight 2-tablespoon servings) / **Per Serving** Calories: 120 Total fat: 10.7g Saturated fat: 1.5g Protein: 0.3g Carbohydrates: 7g Fiber: 0g Cholesterol: 0mg

COOKING TIP

A small lidded jar works perfectly for making and storing a vinaigrette. Just add the ingredients to the jar, put on the lid, and shake. Store in the jar in the refrigerator, bring to room temperature, and shake again to serve.

Lemon Vinaigrette

VEGETARIAN   GLUTEN-FREE   DAIRY-FREE

Prep time: 5 minutes   **Cooking time:** None

This classic French-style vinaigrette is simple to make and extremely versatile. Use it to dress just about any salad of mixed vegetables, chicken, or shrimp. It is also fantastic with salads of cooked grain such as quinoa or brown rice.

- Zest and juice of 2 fresh lemons
- ¼ cup Dijon mustard
- 2 teaspoons honey
- 1 garlic clove, minced
- 2 teaspoons salt
- 1 teaspoon freshly ground black pepper
- ¼ cup olive oil

In a small bowl, add the lemon zest and juice, mustard, honey, garlic, salt, and pepper and whisk to combine. Add the olive oil and whisk until the dressing is emulsified. Vinaigrette can be stored in the refrigerator for up to 1 week. Bring to room temperature, and shake or whisk well before using.

Makes about 1 cup (eight 2-tablespoon servings) / **Per Serving** Calories: 66   Total fat: 6.6g   Saturated fat: 0.9g   Protein: 0.4g   Carbohydrates: 2.2g   Fiber: 0g   Cholesterol: 0mg

> **INGREDIENT VARIATIONS**
>
> This versatile dressing can be flavored in many different ways. Add a tablespoon of fresh herbs such as rosemary, basil, thyme, oregano, or tarragon to create different flavor profiles. And a teaspoon of dried spices such as smoked paprika, cumin, curry powder, or chili powder can give the dressing a whole new taste.

Yogurt Dressing

VEGETARIAN   GLUTEN-FREE

Prep time: 2 minutes   **Cooking time:** None

This simple, creamy dressing is made with rich and tangy yogurt. With only a handful of pantry ingredients, it makes a versatile sauce that can be used to top anything from a green salad to a pita sandwich or Quinoa-Stuffed Peppers (page 141). It also makes a tasty dip for chips or crudités.

- 2 cups plain yogurt
- 2 teaspoons ground cumin
- 2 teaspoons smoked paprika
- 1 teaspoon salt
- ½ teaspoon freshly ground black pepper

In a small bowl, add the yogurt, cumin, paprika, salt, and pepper and stir to combine well. Serve immediately, or store tightly covered in the refrigerator for up to 1 week.

Makes 2 cups (eight ¼-cup servings) / Per Serving Calories: 28   Total fat: 0.8g   Saturated fat: 0.5g   Protein: 3.4g   Carbohydrates: 1.7g   Fiber 0g   Cholesterol: 2mg

Homemade Mayonnaise

VEGETARIAN   DAIRY-FREE   GLUTEN-FREE

Prep time: 5 minutes   **Cooking time:** None

Once you've tried homemade mayonnaise, you'll never go back to the store-bought kind, and not just because it's loaded with additives. Homemade mayonnaise just tastes so much better! This classic version is made of egg yolk and olive oil, with a bit of lemon juice, vinegar, Dijon mustard, and salt for flavor.

- 1 egg yolk
- 1½ teaspoons freshly squeezed lemon juice
- 1 teaspoon white wine vinegar
- ¼ teaspoon Dijon mustard
- ½ teaspoon salt
- ¾ cup olive oil

1. In the bowl of a blender (or food processor), combine the egg yolk, lemon juice, vinegar, mustard, and salt. With the blender running and the lid on, slowly drizzle the oil in through the hole in the lid. Continue blending until all the oil has been added and the mixture is thick.

2. Transfer to a storage container and store, tightly covered, in the refrigerator for up to 3 days.

Makes about ¾ cup (or six 1-tablespoon servings) / **Per Serving** Calories: 113   Total fat: 13g   Saturated fat: 2g   Protein: 0.3g   Carbohydrates: 0.1g   Fiber: 0g   Cholesterol: 18mg

> **COOKING TIP**
>
> If you prefer not to use raw eggs, you can make a cooked version by combining the egg yolk, lemon juice, vinegar, mustard, and salt in the top of a double boiler set over simmering water and whisk just until the mixture begins to thicken. Set the pan in a dish of cold water to stop cooking, and then transfer the mixture to a blender, and proceed with the recipe as written.

Salsa Verde

VEGETARIAN   VEGAN   GLUTEN-FREE   DAIRY-FREE

Prep time: 5 minutes   **Cooking time:** None

Quick and versatile, this Mexican-style green sauce is tangy from tomatillos and lime juice, spicy from the jalapeño peppers, and has a bright herbiness from fresh cilantro. Add a bit of sour cream or yogurt to it and use it as a sauce for Chicken Enchiladas Verdes (page 168) or use it as is to top Grilled Shrimp Tacos with Salsa Verde (page 152). It's also fantastic as a dip for tortilla chips.

- 2 (28-ounce) cans tomatillos, drained
- 2 garlic cloves
- 2 tablespoons olive oil
- 2 jalapeño peppers
- Juice of 1 freshly squeezed lime
- 1½ teaspoons salt
- 2 cups chopped fresh cilantro

In the bowl of a blender (or food processor), add the tomatillos, garlic, olive oil, jalapeño peppers, lime juice, salt, and fresh cilantro and process to a purée. Taste and adjust seasoning if needed. Use immediately, or store in a tightly covered container in the refrigerator for up to 5 days.

Makes about 4 cups (eight ½-cup servings) / **Per Serving** Calories: 97   Total fat: 5.6g   Saturated fat: 12.1g   Protein: 2.6g   Carbohydrates: 12.2g   Fiber: 4g   Cholesterol: 0mg

Fresh Basil Pesto

VEGETARIAN   VEGAN   DAIRY-FREE   GLUTEN-FREE

Prep time: 5 minutes   **Cooking time:** None

Endlessly versatile, fresh basil pesto can be used in a million ways. This version uses nutritional yeast—which can be found in health food and natural foods stores—in place of the traditional Parmesan cheese.

- 3 garlic cloves
- 1/3 cup walnuts
- 2 cups fresh basil leaves
- 2 tablespoons nutritional yeast
- 1/2 cup olive oil
- Salt
- Freshly ground black pepper

1. In the bowl of a food processor (or blender), chop the garlic. Add the walnuts and pulse to chop. Add the basil and process until finely chopped. Add the nutritional yeast and pulse a few times to mix in.

2. With the food processor running, add the olive oil in a thin stream, stopping to scrape down the sides of the bowl as needed. Season with salt and pepper. Serve immediately, or store tightly covered in the refrigerator for up to 1 week or in the freezer for up to 3 months.

Makes about 1 cup (eight 2-tablespoon servings) / **Per Serving** Calories: 152   Total fat: 15.9g   Saturated fat: 2g   Protein: 2.1g   Carbohydrates: 2.2g   Fiber: 1.1g   Cholesterol: 0mg

---

INGREDIENT VARIATIONS

Just about any fresh herb can be used for pesto. Try replacing the basil with cilantro, mint, or parsley. The walnuts, too, can be replaced with pine nuts, pecans, almonds, or peanuts.

Romesco Sauce

VEGETARIAN   VEGAN   GLUTEN-FREE   DAIRY-FREE

Prep time: 5 minutes   **Cooking time:** None

This Spanish roasted red bell pepper sauce is thickened with ground almonds and given an acidic punch from sherry vinegar. Traditionally served as a dipping sauce for grilled prawns, it's also fantastic on roasted or grilled fish or chicken or used as a dip for crudités. If you want to make your own roasted red bell peppers, see the Ingredient Tip on page 189.

- 1 (8-ounce) jar roasted red bell peppers, rinsed and drained
- 1 garlic clove
- ¼ cup almonds
- 1 tablespoon white wine vinegar
- ½ teaspoon salt
- ¼ teaspoon cayenne pepper

In the bowl of a food processor (or blender), add the bell peppers, garlic, almonds, vinegar, salt, and pepper and process to a smooth purée. Serve immediately, or store tightly covered in the refrigerator for up to 1 week.

Makes about 1 cup (four ¼-cup servings) / Per Serving Calories: 45   Total fat: 3.1g   Saturated fat: 0g   Protein: 1.6g   Carbohydrates: 3.4g   Fiber 1.4g   Cholesterol: 0mg

Spicy Tomato Sauce

VEGETARIAN   VEGAN   GLUTEN-FREE   DAIRY-FREE

Prep time: 10 minutes   **Cooking time:** 1 hour 10 minutes

In any supermarket, you'll find dozens of kinds of jarred tomato sauce. Many of them are even organic or all-natural, but nearly every one contains something—refined sugar, artificial colors or flavors, excess sodium, or preservatives—that you are trying to avoid with clean eating. Make a giant batch of your own and you'll have delicious, clean tomato sauce at the ready at all times.

- 2 tablespoons olive oil
- 3 medium onions, chopped
- 4 garlic cloves, minced
- 2 tablespoons balsamic vinegar
- 3 (28-ounce) cans crushed tomatoes with their juice
- 2 teaspoons dried oregano
- 1 teaspoon cayenne pepper
- 1 teaspoon salt
- 1 teaspoon freshly ground black pepper

1. In a large stockpot, heat the olive oil over medium-high heat. Add the onion, and cook for about 5 minutes, stirring frequently, until soft. Add the garlic and cook, stirring constantly, for 1 minute.

2. Stir in the balsamic vinegar and then the tomatoes, oregano, cayenne pepper, salt, and black pepper. Bring the mixture to a boil, and then reduce the heat to low and simmer, uncovered, stirring occasionally, for about 1 hour until the sauce is thickened.

3. Let cool and then transfer to storage containers and store in the refrigerator for up to 1 week or in the freezer for up to 3 months.

Makes about 9 cups (eighteen ½-cup servings) / Per Serving Calories: 114   Total fat: 2.4g   Saturated fat: 0g   Protein: 5.1g   Carbohydrates: 19g   Fiber: 7g   Cholesterol: 0mg

Chicken Broth

GLUTEN-FREE   DAIRY-FREE

Prep time: 5 minutes   **Cooking time:** 4 hours

Chicken broth is one of the most useful staples to have around for home cooking. To make broth with intense flavor, return the broth to the stockpot after straining it, bring it to a boil, then simmer for 2 to 3 hours to reduce it.

- 2 tablespoons olive oil
- Carcass of 1 whole cooked chicken
- 1 onion, diced
- 2 carrots, diced
- 3 celery stalks, diced
- 2 garlic cloves, minced
- 2 bay leaves
- 1 teaspoon salt
- ½ teaspoon freshly ground black pepper
- Water to cover (about 4 to 6 quarts)

1. In a large stockpot, heat the oil over medium-high heat. Add the chicken carcass and cook for about 5 minutes, stirring occasionally, until it begins to brown. Add the onion, carrots, celery, garlic, bay leaves, salt, pepper, and water and bring to a boil. Reduce the heat to low and simmer, uncovered, for at least 4 hours, occasionally skimming off any foam that comes to the surface.

2. Strain the stock through a fine-meshed sieve or a cheesecloth-lined colander and discard the solids. Store tightly covered in the refrigerator for up to 3 days or in the freezer for up to 3 months.

Makes about 2 quarts (eight 1-cup servings) / Per Serving Calories: 38   Total fat: 1.4g   Saturated fat: 0g   Protein: 4.8g   Carbohydrates: 0.9g   Fiber: 0g   Cholesterol: 1mg

Vegetable Broth

VEGETARIAN   VEGAN   GLUTEN-FREE   DAIRY-FREE

Prep time: 5 minutes   **Cooking time:** 4 hours

Vegetable broth is a handy staple to have in your refrigerator or freezer. Use it to make vegetarian soups, sauces, stews, and chili. This is a basic vegetable broth, but you can save all sorts of vegetable scraps—corn cobs, leek trimmings, spinach stems, etc.—until you're ready to make it, and use them to add even more flavor. Just toss them in frozen, along with the carrots and celery.

- 2 tablespoons olive oil
- 2 onions, diced
- 4 carrots, diced
- 6 celery stalks, diced
- 2 cloves garlic, minced
- 2 bay leaves
- 1 teaspoon salt
- ½ teaspoon freshly ground black pepper
- Water to cover (about 4 to 6 quarts)

1. In a large stockpot, heat the oil over medium-high heat. Add the onions and cook for about 5 minutes, stirring occasionally, until softened. Add the carrots, celery, garlic, bay leaves, salt, pepper, and water and bring to a boil. Reduce the heat to low and simmer, uncovered, for at least 4 hours.

2. Strain the stock through a fine-meshed sieve or a cheesecloth-lined colander and discard the solids. Store in the refrigerator tightly covered for up to 3 days or in the freezer for up to 3 months.

Makes about 2 quarts (eight 1-cup servings) / **Per Serving** Calories: 38   Total fat: 1.4g   Saturated fat: 0g   Protein: 4.8g   Carbohydrates: 0.9g   Fiber: 0g   Cholesterol: 0mg

Cashew Cheese

VEGETARIAN VEGAN GLUTEN-FREE DAIRY-FREE

Prep time: 10 minutes (plus 30 minutes to soak the cashews)   **Cooking time:** None

Cashew cheese is a rich, creamy, dairy-free cheese substitute. It's made of raw cashews with Dijon mustard, garlic, lemon juice, vinegar, and, the secret ingredient, nutritional yeast, added for flavor. Nutritional yeast can be found in any health food or natural foods store and it is what provides the fermented flavor you expect from cheese. You can use Cashew Cheese when you'd use regular cheese—spread it on toast, pizza, or celery sticks. Use it in tacos, as a dip, or in sandwiches. The possibilities are endless.

- 1 cup cashews
- ¼ cup water
- ¼ cup nutritional yeast
- 2 tablespoons freshly squeezed lemon juice
- 2 garlic cloves
- 2 tablespoons white wine vinegar
- 1 tablespoon Dijon mustard
- ¼ teaspoon salt

In the bowl of a blender (or food processor), add the cashews, water, yeast, lemon juice, garlic, vinegar, mustard, and salt, and process until the mixture is smooth and creamy. Serve immediately, or store, tightly covered, in the refrigerator for up to 1 week.

Makes about 1½ cups (twenty 2-tablespoon servings) / Per Serving Calories: 80 Total fat: 5.5g   Saturated fat: 1.1g   Protein: 3.4g   Carbohydrates: 5.6g   Fiber 1.2g   Cholesterol: 0mg

Homemade Almond Milk

VEGETARIAN   VEGAN   GLUTEN-FREE   DAIRY-FREE

Prep time: 10 minutes (plus overnight to soak the almonds)   **Cooking time:** None

Store-bought almond milk often contains sweeteners or other undesirable additives. The almonds should be soaked for at least 8 to 12 hours, and they can be soaked for as long as 2 days. The longer you soak them, the creamier the resulting almond milk will be. If you like your almond milk with a touch of sweetness, feel free to add a little honey or other natural sweetener.

1 cup raw almonds
2 cups water, plus more for the almonds

1. In a medium bowl, put the almonds and add cold water to cover by about 1 inch. Let the almonds soak overnight uncovered.

2. Drain the almonds, discard the soaking water, and rinse them thoroughly with cold water.

3. In the bowl of a blender (or food processor), add the almonds and the 2 cups water and blend at high speed for 2 minutes. Scrape down the sides of the bowl, as needed, and blend for 2 to 3 minutes more, until the nuts are finely ground and the liquid is white.

4. Line a colander with a fine-mesh nut milk bag or a square of cheesecloth, and place it over a bowl. Pour the puréed almond mixture into the nut milk bag, letting the liquid run through into the bowl. Squeeze the bag to get as much of the liquid out as you can. Serve immediately.

5. Almond milk can be stored in a tightly covered jar in the refrigerator for up to 2 days.

Makes about 2 cups (sixteen ½-cup servings) / Per Serving Calories: 137   Total fat: 11.9g   Saturated fat: 1.5g   Protein: 5g   Carbohydrates: 5.1g   Fiber: 3g   Cholesterol: 0mg

Whipped Coconut Cream

VEGETARIAN   GLUTEN-FREE   DAIRY-FREE

Prep time: 10 minutes   **Cooking time:** None

Nothing compares to a fluffy dollop of sweetened whipped cream atop a serving of baked dessert. Thanks to this recipe, you can enjoy a dairy-free version that's just as rich and delicious. Use it to embellish any baked dessert from Apple Crisp with Fresh Ginger (page 200) to Banana Chocolate Tart (page 204) or as a dip for fresh strawberries.

- 1 cup coconut cream
- 2 tablespoons honey (or maple syrup, for a vegan version)
- ½ teaspoon vanilla extract

In a large bowl and using a hand mixer set on high speed, add the coconut cream and whip it for about 5 to 7 minutes until it becomes fluffy and forms soft peaks. Add the honey (or maple syrup) and vanilla and beat just to incorporate. Serve immediately, or store in the refrigerator in a tightly covered container for up to 2 days.

Makes 8 servings / Per Serving Calories: 86   Total fat: 7.2g   Saturated fat: 6.3g   Protein: 0.7g   Carbohydrates: 6g   Fiber: 0.7g   Cholesterol: 0mg

INGREDIENT TIP

If you can't find coconut cream, you can use regular, full-fat coconut milk. Place a 14-ounce can of coconut milk in the refrigerator overnight. Open the can without shaking it or turning it over. The contents of the can will have separated and the thick cream will have risen to the top. Scoop the thick cream out of the can (you should have about 1 cup) and proceed with the recipe as written. Save the remaining coconut milk for another use.

Appendix A 10 Tips for Dining Out

Dining out can present a challenge when you are following any eating plan, and it can be especially difficult with clean eating since many of the ingredients you are trying to avoid can be hidden in restaurant dishes. Here are a few ideas to help you get through a restaurant meal with your clean eating status intact.

1. **Believe that it's possible to eat clean while dining out.** Don't assume that there won't be anything clean for you to eat when you dine out and use that as an excuse to toss your clean eating plans out the window. These days, as more and more restaurants embrace the back-to-basics, farm-to-table approach to food, there are more options than you might expect.

2. **Choose wisely.** If possible, choose a restaurant or style of cuisine that is likely to provide clean options. Look for a restaurant that serves grilled fish, chicken, or meat; salads; and lots of vegetables. Indian or Middle Eastern restaurants, for instance, often feature fresh dishes with lots of vegetables, legumes, and grilled meats. In Chinese restaurants, avoid ordering sauced dishes, which are often loaded with sugar and maybe other additives like monosodium glutamate (MSG).

3. **Plan ahead.** If you can't choose the restaurant, try to check the menu ahead of time to see if there are any clean options. If you can't tell from the menu, call and ask.

4. **Don't be afraid to ask for changes.** If a restaurant serves grilled chicken or ribs topped with sugar-heavy barbecue sauce, ask if you can have the sauce left off. Likewise, if the broccoli comes drenched in cheese sauce. If side dishes like pasta or French fries are included with your dish, ask them to substitute cooked vegetables or salad instead.

5. **Order wisely.** Choose steamed, poached, grilled, roasted, or broiled dishes over fried or sautéed, which are far more likely to contain forbidden ingredients.

6. **Skip white rice and white pasta.** If you can't substitute vegetables for refined-carbohydrate foods like pasta and white rice, ask if you can substitute brown rice or whole-wheat pasta, or ask for these items to simply be left off your plate.

7. **Avoid foods with sauce.** Sauces are delicious, but they often contain sugar, carbohydrates, and other undesirable ingredients. Your safest bet is to avoid foods that come topped with lots of sauce. Some exceptions are fresh salsas, if they are made only of fresh fruits, vegetables, and spices. Vinaigrettes, too, can be safe, but do ask about the ingredients since many contain sugar or thickeners.

8. **Be cautious with condiments.** Sugar, refined grains, artificial flavors and colors, preservatives, and other additives hide in condiments like relish, ketchup, and barbecue sauce, so be sure to check the labels and find alternatives wherever necessary.

9. **Stick to water.** Most restaurant beverages are on the list of foods to avoid, so a good choice is to stick to water. Ask for sparkling water with a wedge of lemon or lime, if you like.

10. **Skip dessert.** Sadly, restaurant desserts are pretty much always made with sugar and refined flour. Wait until you get home and then have fruit or a homemade dessert that fits the clean eating plan.

Appendix B   Conversion Tables

Volume Equivalents (Liquid)

U.S. Standard	U.S. Standard (ounces)	Metric (approximate)
2 tablespoons	1 fl. oz.	30 mL
¼ cup	2 fl. oz.	60 mL
½ cup	4 fl. oz.	120 mL
1 cup	8 fl. oz.	240 mL
1½ cups	12 fl. oz.	355 mL
2 cups or 1 pint	16 fl. oz.	475 mL
4 cups or 1 quart	32 fl. oz.	1 L
1 gallon	128 fl. oz.	4 L

Oven Temperatures

Fahrenheit (F)	Celsius (C) (approximate)
250	120
300	150
325	165
350	180
375	190
400	200
425	220
450	230

Volume Equivalents (Dry)

U.S. Standard	Metric (approximate)
⅛ teaspoon	0.5 mL
¼ teaspoon	1 mL
½ teaspoon	2 mL
¾ teaspoon	4 mL
1 teaspoon	5 mL
1 tablespoon	15 mL
¼ cup	59 mL
⅓ cup	79 mL
½ cup	118 mL
⅔ cup	156 mL
¾ cup	177 mL
1 cup	235 mL
2 cups or 1 pint	475 mL
3 cups	700 mL
4 cups or 1 quart	1 L
½ gallon	2 L
1 gallon	4 L

Weight Equivalents

U.S. Standard	Metric (approximate)
½ ounce	15 g
1 ounce	30 g
2 ounces	60 g
4 ounces	115 g
8 ounces	225 g
12 ounces	340 g
16 ounces or 1 pound	455 g

Resources

The clean eating lifestyle is enjoying a surge in popularity. Lots of websites and magazines have popped up to provide information to those who wish to adopt the lifestyle. There are also numerous healthful cooking and lifestyle magazines and websites that provide great recipes and tips that can help you stay the clean eating course. Many Paleo diet–oriented websites and magazines, too, provide recipes and advice that fit the clean eating lifestyle.

Magazines

These print magazines also have websites where you can find the recipes printed in the magazines.

Clean Eating magazine   www.cleaneatingmag.com
Cooking Light magazine   www.cookinglight.com
Eating Well magazine   www.eatingwell.com
Fitness magazine   www.fitnessmagazine.com
Oxygen magazine   www.oxygenmag.com

Websites

These websites provide information and advice on the clean eating lifestyle as well as recipes.

Busy But Healthy   www.busybuthealthy.com
Clean and Delicious   www.cleananddelicious.com
The Gracious Pantry   www.thegraciouspantry.com
He and She Eat Clean   www.heandsheeatclean.com
The Naked Kitchen   www.thenakedkitchen.com

References

American Cancer Society. "Common Questions About Diet and Cancer." Accessed May 5, 2014. www.cancer.org/healthy/eathealthygetactive/acsguidelinesonnutritionphysicalactivityforcancerprevention/acs-guidelines-on-nutrition-and-physical-activity-for-cancer-prevention-common-questions.

Brandt, Frederic, MD. "Face the Facts About Sugar." *Prevention* magazine. Accessed June 4, 2014. www.prevention.com/beauty/beauty/how-sugar-ages-your-skin.

Cassetty, Samantha B., MS, RD, and Delia Hammock, MS, RD. "Best Anti-Aging Foods." WebMD. Accessed May 6, 2014. www.webmd.com/diet/features/best-anti-aging-foods.

Center for Science in the Public Interest. "Coconut Oil." Accessed June 7, 2014. www.cspinet.org/nah/articles/coconut-oil.html.

Eatright.org. "Family Nutrition and Physical Activity Report." Accessed June 4, 2014. www.eatright.org/foundation/fnpa/.

Environmental Working Group. "All 48 Fruits and Vegetables with Pesticide Residue." Accessed May 6, 2014. www.ewg.org/foodnews/list.php.

Gorman, Rachael Moeller. "Fresh vs. Frozen Vegetables: Are We Giving Up Nutrition for Convenience?" *Eating Well*. Accessed May 9, 2014. www.eatingwell.com/nutrition_health/nutrition_news_information/fresh_vs_frozen_vegetables_are_we_giving_up_nutrition_fo.

Harvard.edu. "Microwave Cooking and Nutrition." Accessed May 9, 2014. www.health.harvard.edu/fhg/updates/Microwave-cooking-and-nutrition.shtml.

Harvard School of Public Health Nutrition Source. "Fats and Cholesterol: Out with the Bad, In with the Good." Accessed May 5, 2014. www.hsph.harvard.edu/nutritionsource/fats-full-story/.

Lester, Gene, PhD. "Vegetable Debate: Fresh, Frozen, or Canned?" RD411. Accessed June 7, 2014. www.nutrition411.com/patient-education-materials/fruits-and-vegetables/item/28481-vegetable-debate-fresh-frozen-or-canned/.

LoGiudice, Pina, ND, Siobhan Bleakney, ND, and Peter Bongiorno, ND. "The Surprising Health Benefits of Coconut Oil." *Dr. Oz*. Accessed May 12, 2014. www.doctoroz.com/videos/surprising-health-benefits-coconut-oil.

Mayo Clinic. "Depression." Accessed May 5, 2014. www.mayoclinic.org/diseases-conditions/depression/basics/definition/con-20032977.

Mayo Clinic. "Nutrition and Healthy Eating." Accessed May 6, 2014. www.mayoclinic.org/healthy-living/nutrition-and-healthy-eating/in-depth/fiber/art-20043983.

Moyad, Mark, MD. "Vitamin C Dietary Supplements: An Objective Review of the Clinical Evidence, Part I." *Seminars in Preventive and Alternative Medicine* vol. 3, no. 1: pages 25–35.

Tsikitis, V. L., J. E. Albina, and J. S. Reichner. "Beta-Glucan Affects Leukocyte Navigation in a Complex Chemotactic Gradient." *Surgery*. August 2004.

WebMD. "Aging Well." Accessed June 4, 2014. www.webmd.com/healthy-aging/features/aging-well-eating-right-for-longevity.

WebMD. "The Many Benefits of Breakfast." Accessed May 6, 2014. www.webmd.com/diet/features/many-benefits-breakfast.

Recipe Index

A
Apple Crisp with Fresh Ginger, 200–201
Apple Walnut Bars, 115

B
Bacon-Crusted Mini Quiches with Mushrooms and Greens, 84–85
Bacon-Wrapped Meatloaf, 188–189
Balsamic-Glazed Wild Salmon with Garlicky Sautéed Spinach, 157–158
Balsamic-Roasted Vegetables with Quinoa, 139–140
Balsamic Vinaigrette, 214
Banana Blueberry Whole-Grain Pancakes, 74–75
Banana Chocolate Tart, 204–205
Banana Maple Nut "Ice Cream," 197
Banana Nut Bread, 116–117
Basil Garlic Zucchini Chips, 122
Berry Crumb Cake, 202–203
Breakfast Tacos with Green Chiles, Goat Cheese, and Salsa Verde, 79–80
Brown Rice and Black Bean Salad with Spinach and Lemon Vinaigrette, 97
Brussels Sprouts and Chickpea Salad with Dried Cranberries, 95
Brussels Sprouts Hash with Caramelized Onions and Poached Eggs, 148–149

C
Caprese Salad with Balsamic Vinaigrette, 90
Cashew Cheese, 224
Chicken and White Bean Chili, 175–176
Chicken Broth, 222
Chicken Enchiladas Verdes with Goat Cheese, 168–169
Chickpea Tostadas with Cashew Cheese, 133–134
Cocoa Almond Pudding, 198
Creamy Peanut Butter–Yogurt Dip, 119
Curried Chicken Salad Lettuce Wraps with Homemade Mayonnaise, 103

E
Egg Salad Sandwich with Greek Yogurt and Dill, 102

F
Fresh Basil Pesto, 219
Fresh Herb Frittata with Peas, Bacon, and Feta Cheese, 88–89

G
Garden Salad with Chicken and Balsamic Vinaigrette, 100
Garlic-Broiled Shrimp and Peppers over Quinoa, 154–155
Ginger Berry Smoothie, 60
Goat Cheese and Spinach–Stuffed Pork Chops, 181–182
Grilled Pineapple and Pork Skewers, 183
Grilled Shrimp Tacos with Salsa Verde and Spicy Slaw, 152–153
Guacamole, 212

H
Homemade Almond Milk, 225
Homemade Cinnamon Granola, 61–62
Homemade Mayonnaise, 217
Honey Sesame Crackers, 118

I
Italian Fish Stew, 163

K
Korean Pork Lettuce Wraps with Fresh Herbs, 105
Korean Stir-Fried Pork with Brown Rice, 184–185

L
Lamb Loin Chops with Yogurt-Mint Sauce, 179–180
Lemon Vinaigrette, 215

M
Mediterranean Chickpea Salad with Red Bell Peppers and Feta Cheese, 94
Mini Cheesecakes in Caramel Sauce, 208–209
Molten Chocolate Cakes, 206

N
No-Bake Coconut Granola Bars, 63–64

O

Oven-Baked Sweet Potato Fries, 123
Oven-Roasted Monkfish and Asparagus with Romesco Sauce, 160
Overnight Cinnamon Oatmeal, 65

P

Peanut Butter Energy Bites, 113
Peanut Butter Oatmeal Cookies, 199
Pesto White Bean Spread, 124
Pico de Gallo, 213
Pineapple Coconut Trail Mix, 112
Poached Eggs and Asparagus on Whole-Grain Toast, 82–83
Poached Eggs in Spicy Tomato Sauce, 81
Pork Fried Brown Rice with Pineapple and Cashews, 186–187
Protein-Packed Freezer Waffles (or Pancakes), 66–67
Pumpkin and Chickpea Curry, 132

Q

Quinoa Fried "Rice" with Flank Steak and Peas, 192–193
Quinoa Salad with Cannellini Beans, Tomatoes, and Lemon Vinaigrette, 96
Quinoa-Stuffed Peppers with Black Beans and Yogurt Dressing, 141–142

R

Red Pepper, Spinach, and Goat Cheese Frittata Bites, 76
Red Snapper with Spiced Pumpkin Seed Butter, 159
Rich Chocolate Fudge, 207
Risotto with Mushrooms and Peas, 146–147
Roasted Butternut Squash and Black Bean Burritos with Goat Cheese, 137–138
Roasted Butternut Squash Salad with Goat Cheese, Walnuts, and Balsamic Vinaigrette, 92–93
Roasted Chicken and Vegetables, 166–167
Roasted Chicken Breasts with Mustard and Greens, 172–173
Roasted Vegetable Pitas with Pesto Mayonnaise, 101
Romesco Sauce, 220

S

Salsa Verde, 218
Scrambled Egg, Goat Cheese, and Cherry Tomato Pita Sandwich, 77–78
Seared Ahi Tuna with Chili-Lime Aioli, 156
Sesame-Soy Marinated Flank Steak with Wasabi-Spiked Cauliflower Purée, 190–191
Shrimp Salad over Greens with Yogurt Dressing, 98
Smoky Red Lentil Soup with Greens, 106–107
Smoky-Sweet Chili Almonds, 121
Soy-Glaze Cod with Japanese-Style Pickled Cucumber, 161–162
Spiced Chicken Wraps with Yogurt Dressing and Fresh Mint, 104
Spiced Roasted Chickpeas, 120
Spicy Black Bean Soup with Vegetables, 108–109
Spicy Southwestern Corn and Bean Salad, 91
Spicy Tomato Sauce, 221
Spinach and White Bean Enchiladas with Cashew Cheese, 135–136
Spinach Salad with Chicken and Sun-Dried Tomatoes and Basil Vinaigrette, 99
Stacked Eggplant Parmesan, 128–129
Sweet Quinoa Breakfast Cups, 72–73

T

Tandoori-Spiced Chicken Breast with Crisp Cucumber Salad, 170–171
Thai-Style Curried Chicken Burgers, 174
Tropical Sweet Bars, 114
Turkey Meatballs with Whole-Wheat Spaghetti and Spicy Tomato Sauce, 177–178

V

Vegetable Broth, 223
Vegetable Stew, 144–145
Vegetarian Chili with Pinto Beans, 130–131

W

Whipped Coconut Cream, 226
Whole-Wheat Blueberry Muffins with Cinnamon-Sugar Topping, 70–71
Whole-Wheat Maple Cinnamon Rolls, 68–69
Whole-Wheat Pasta with Chickpeas and Spicy Tomato Sauce, 143

Y

Yogurt Blueberry Ice Pops, 196
Yogurt Dressing, 216

Index

A

Almond flour, 13
   Bacon-Wrapped Meatloaf, 188–189
   Banana Chocolate Tart, 204–205
   Berry Crumb Cake, 202–203
   Stacked Eggplant Parmesan, 128–129

Almond milk
   Berry Crumb Cake, 202–203
   Cocoa Almond Pudding, 198
   Fresh Herb Frittata with Peas, Bacon, and Feta Cheese, 88–89
   Ginger Berry Smoothie, 60
   Overnight Cinnamon Oatmeal, 65
   Red Pepper, Spinach, and Goat Cheese Frittata Bites, 76
   Rich Chocolate Fudge, 207
   Scrambled Egg, Goat Cheese, and Cherry Tomato Pita Sandwich, 77–78
   Whole-Wheat Blueberry Muffins with Cinnamon-Sugar Topping, 70–71
   Whole-Wheat Maple Cinnamon Rolls, 68–69

Almonds
   Homemade Almond Milk, 225
   Homemade Cinnamon Granola, 61–62
   No-Bake Coconut Granola Bars, 63–64
   Pineapple Coconut Trail Mix, 112
   Romesco Sauce, 220
   Smoky-Sweet Chili Almonds, 121

Amy's, 19
Antioxidants, 3–4
Apples
   Apple Crisp with Fresh Ginger, 200–201
   Apple Walnut Bars, 115
   Curried Chicken Salad Lettuce Wraps with Homemade Mayonnaise, 103
   Sweet Quinoa Breakfast Cups, 72–73

Arborio rice
   Risotto with Mushrooms and Peas, 146–147

Asparagus
   Oven-Roasted Monkfish and Asparagus with Romesco Sauce, 160
   Poached Eggs and Asparagus on Whole-Grain Toast, 82–83

Avocados
   Garden Salad with Chicken and Balsamic Vinaigrette, 100
   Guacamole, 212

B

Bacon
   Bacon-Crusted Mini Quiches with Mushrooms and Greens, 84–85
   Bacon-Wrapped Meatloaf, 188–189
   Fresh Herb Frittata with Peas, Bacon, and Feta Cheese, 88–89

Baking, 25
Balanced meals, eating, 5
Balsamic-Glazed Wild Salmon with Garlicky Sautéed Spinach, 157–158
Balsamic-Roasted Vegetables with Quinoa, 139–140
Balsamic Vinaigrette, 214
   Caprese Salad with Balsamic Vinaigrette, 90
   Garden Salad with Chicken and Balsamic Vinaigrette, 100
   Roasted Butternut Squash Salad with Goat Cheese, Walnuts, and Balsamic Vinaigrette, 92–93
   Spinach Salad with Chicken and Sun-Dried Tomatoes and Basil Vinaigrette, 99

Bananas
   Banana Blueberry Whole-Grain Pancakes, 74–75
   Banana Chocolate Tart, 204–205
   Banana Maple Nut "Ice Cream," 197
   Banana Nut Bread, 116–117
   Ginger Berry Smoothie, 60

Barley, 2
Bars. *See also* Cookies
   Apple Walnut Bars, 115
   Tropical Sweet Bars, 114

Basil
   Basil Garlic Zucchini Chips, 122
   Caprese Salad with Balsamic Vinaigrette, 90

Fresh Basil Pesto, 219
Korean Pork Lettuce Wraps with Fresh Herbs, 105
Poached Eggs in Spicy Tomato Sauce, 81
Spinach Salad with Chicken and Sun-Dried Tomatoes and Basil Vinaigrette, 99
Whole-Wheat Pasta with Chickpeas and Spicy Tomato Sauce, 143
B-complex vitamins, 2
Beans. *See* Black beans; Cannellini beans; Green beans; Pinto beans
Beef. *See also* Ground beef
Quinoa Fried "Rice" with Flank Steak and Peas, 192–193
Sesame-Soy Marinated Flank Steak with Wasabi-Spiked Cauliflower Purée, 190–191
Bell peppers. *See* Red bell peppers; Yellow bell peppers
Berry Crumb Cake, 202–203
Beta-glucans, 2
Beverages, high-calorie, 11
Black beans
Brown Rice and Black Bean Salad with Spinach and Lemon Vinaigrette, 97
Quinoa-Stuffed Peppers with Black Beans and Yogurt Dressing, 141–142
Roasted Butternut Squash and Black Bean Burritos with Goat Cheese, 137–138
Spicy Black Bean Soup with Vegetables, 108–109
Spicy Southwestern Corn and Bean Salad, 91
Blood sugar, regulating your, 2
Blueberries
Banana Blueberry Whole-Grain Pancakes, 74–75

Berry Crumb Cake, 202–203
Whole-Wheat Blueberry Muffins with Cinnamon-Sugar Topping, 70–71
Yogurt Blueberry Ice Pops, 196
Boiling, 26
BPA (bisphenol-A), 19
Braising, 26
Breads, Banana Nut, 116–117
Breakfast, 59–85
Bacon-Crusted Mini Quiches with Mushrooms and Greens, 84–85
Banana Blueberry Whole-Grain Pancakes, 74–75
Breakfast Tacos with Green Chiles, Goat Cheese, and Salsa Verde, 79–80
Ginger Berry Smoothie, 60
Homemade Cinnamon Granola, 61–62
No-Bake Coconut Granola Bars, 63–64
Overnight Cinnamon Oatmeal, 65
Poached Eggs and Asparagus on Whole-Grain Toast, 82–83
Poached Eggs in Spicy Tomato Sauce, 81
Protein-Packed Freezer Waffles (or Pancakes), 66–67
Red Pepper, Spinach, and Goat Cheese Frittata Bites, 76
Scrambled Egg, Goat Cheese, and Cherry Tomato Pita Sandwich, 77–78
skipping, 15
Sweet Quinoa Breakfast Cups, 72–73
Whole-Wheat Blueberry Muffins with Cinnamon-Sugar Topping, 70–71

Whole-Wheat Maple Cinnamon Rolls, 68–69
Brown rice
Brown Rice and Black Bean Salad with Spinach and Lemon Vinaigrette, 97
Korean Stir-Fried Pork with Brown Rice, 184–185
Pork Fried Brown Rice with Pineapple and Cashews, 186–187
Brussels sprouts
Brussels Sprouts and Chickpea Salad with Dried Cranberries, 95
Brussels Sprouts Hash with Caramelized Onions and Poached Eggs, 148–149
Burgers, Thai-Style Curried Chicken, 174
Butternut squash
Roasted Butternut Squash and Black Bean Burritos with Goat Cheese, 137–138
Roasted Butternut Squash Salad with Goat Cheese, Walnuts, and Balsamic Vinaigrette, 92–93

C

Cabbage
Grilled Shrimp Tacos with Salsa Verde and Spicy Slaw, 152–153
Calorie counting, 6
Cannellini beans
Chicken and White Bean Chili, 175–176
Pesto White Bean Spread, 124
Quinoa Salad with Cannellini Beans, Tomatoes, and Lemon Vinaigrette, 96
Spinach and White Bean Enchiladas with Cashew Cheese, 135–136
Canning process, 19

Canola oil, 14
Caprese Salad with Balsamic Vinaigrette, 90
Cardiovascular health, improving, 3
Carrots
　Chicken and White Bean Chili, 175–176
　Chicken Broth, 222
　Korean Pork Lettuce Wraps with Fresh Herbs, 105
　Quinoa Fried "Rice" with Flank Steak and Peas, 192–193
　Roasted Chicken and Vegetables, 166–167
　Smoky Red Lentil Soup with Greens, 106–107
　Spicy Black Bean Soup with Vegetables, 108–109
　Vegetable Broth, 223
　Vegetable Stew, 144–145
　Vegetarian Chili with Pinto Beans, 130–131
Cashew Cheese, 224
　Chickpea Tostadas with Cashew Cheese, 133–134
　Spinach and White Bean Enchiladas with Cashew Cheese, 135–136
Cashews
　Cashew Cheese, 224
　Pork Fried Brown Rice with Pineapple and Cashews, 186–187
　Tropical Sweet Bars, 114
Cauliflower
　Sesame-Soy Marinated Flank Steak with Wasabi-Spiked Cauliflower Purée, 190–191
Celery
　Chicken Broth, 222
　Vegetable Broth, 223
Cheese. See Cashew Cheese; Feta cheese; Goat cheese; Mozzarella cheese

Cherry tomatoes
　Brown Rice and Black Bean Salad with Spinach and Lemon Vinaigrette, 97
　Scrambled Egg, Goat Cheese, and Cherry Tomato Pita Sandwich, 77–78
　Shrimp Salad over Greens with Yogurt Dressing, 98
　Spinach Salad with Chicken and Sun-Dried Tomatoes and Basil Vinaigrette, 99
Chicken
　Chicken and White Bean Chili, 175–176
　Chicken Broth, 222
　Chicken Enchiladas Verdes with Goat Cheese, 168–169
　Curried Chicken Salad Lettuce Wraps with Homemade Mayonnaise, 103
　Garden Salad with Chicken and Balsamic Vinaigrette, 100
　Roasted Chicken and Vegetables, 166–167
　Roasted Chicken Breasts with Mustard and Greens, 172–173
　Spiced Chicken Wraps with Yogurt Dressing and Fresh Mint, 104
　Spinach Salad with Chicken and Sun-Dried Tomatoes and Basil Vinaigrette, 99
　Tandoori-Spiced Chicken Breast with Crisp Cucumber Salad, 170–171
　Thai-Style Curried Chicken Burgers, 174
Chicken Broth, 222
　Chicken and White Bean Chili, 175–176

Chickpea flour, 13
Chickpeas
　Brussels Sprouts and Chickpea Salad with Dried Cranberries, 95
　Chickpea Tostadas with Cashew Cheese, 133–134
　Mediterranean Chickpea Salad with Red Bell Peppers and Feta Cheese, 94
　Pumpkin and Chickpea Curry, 132
　Spiced Roasted Chickpeas, 120
　Whole-Wheat Pasta with Chickpeas and Spicy Tomato Sauce, 143
Chiles
　Breakfast Tacos with Green Chiles, Goat Cheese, and Salsa Verde, 79–80
　Chicken and White Bean Chili, 175–176
Chili
　Chicken and White Bean Chili, 175–176
　Vegetarian Chili with Pinto Beans, 130–131
Cholesterol, lowering your, 3
Cilantro
　Chicken Enchiladas Verdes with Goat Cheese, 168–169
　Grilled Shrimp Tacos with Salsa Verde and Spicy Slaw, 152–153
　Pico de Gallo, 213
　Salsa Verde, 218
　Spicy Southwestern Corn and Bean Salad, 91
　Spinach and White Bean Enchiladas with Cashew Cheese, 135–136
　Thai-Style Curried Chicken Burgers, 174

Cinnamon
- Apple Walnut Bars, 115
- Banana Nut Bread, 116–117
- Berry Crumb Cake, 202–203
- Homemade Cinnamon Granola, 61–62
- No-Bake Coconut Granola Bars, 63–64
- Overnight Cinnamon Oatmeal, 65
- Peanut Butter Oatmeal Cookies, 199
- Smoky Red Lentil Soup with Greens, 106–107
- Sweet Quinoa Breakfast Cups, 72–73
- Whole-Wheat Blueberry Muffins with Cinnamon-Sugar Topping, 70–71
- Whole-Wheat Maple Cinnamon Rolls, 68–69

Clean eating
- comparing with paleo diet, 4
- costs of, 14
- FAQs on, 13–15
- principles of, 5–6
- reasons for choosing, 1–4
- time needed for, 13
- tips for making it work, 27–29

Clean fifteen, 21

Cocoa powder
- Banana Chocolate Tart, 204–205
- Cocoa Almond Pudding, 198
- Molten Chocolate Cakes, 206
- Rich Chocolate Fudge, 207

Coconut
- Homemade Cinnamon Granola, 61–62
- No-Bake Coconut Granola Bars, 63–64
- Peanut Butter Energy Bites, 113
- Pineapple Coconut Trail Mix, 112
- Rich Chocolate Fudge, 207
- Tropical Sweet Bars, 114

Coconut Cream, Whipped, 226
Coconut flour, 13
Coconut oil, 23

Banana Chocolate Tart, 204–205
Banana Nut Bread, 116–117
Berry Crumble Cake, 202–203
Honey Sesame Crackers, 118
Molten Chocolate Cakes, 206
Protein-Packed Freezer Waffles (or Pancakes), 66–67
Whole-Wheat Maple Cinnamon Rolls, 68–69

Coconut sugar
- Apple Crisp with Fresh Ginger, 200–201
- Berry Crumble Cake, 202–203
- Mini Cheesecakes in Caramel Sauce, 208–209
- Molten Chocolate Cakes, 206
- Oven-Baked Sweet Potato Fries, 123
- Peanut Butter Oatmeal Cookies, 199
- Whole-Wheat Blueberry Muffins with Cinnamon-Sugar Topping, 70–71

Cod
- Italian Fish Stew, 163
- Soy-Glazed Cod with Japanese-Style Pickled Cucumber, 161–162

Conversion tables, 229
Cookies. *See also* Bars
- Peanut Butter Oatmeal Cookies, 199

Cooking methods, 25–27

Corn
- Spicy Southwestern Corn and Bean Salad, 91
- Spinach and White Bean Enchiladas with Cashew Cheese, 135–136

Cranberries
- Brussels Sprouts and Chickpea Salad with Dried Cranberries, 95
- No-Bake Coconut Granola Bars, 63–64

Cream cheese
- Mini Cheesecakes in Caramel Sauce, 208–209

Creamy Peanut Butter–Yogurt Dip, 119

Cucumbers
- Brown Rice and Black Bean Salad with Spinach and Lemon Vinaigrette, 97
- Korean Pork Lettuce Wraps with Fresh Herbs, 105
- Mediterranean Chickpea Salad with Red Bell Peppers and Feta Cheese, 94
- Shrimp Salad over Greens with Yogurt Dressing, 98
- Soy-Glazed Cod with Japanese-Style Pickled Cucumber, 161–162
- Spiced Chicken Wraps with Yogurt Dressing and Fresh Mint, 104
- Tandoori-Spiced Chicken Breast with Crisp Cucumber Salad, 170–171

Curried Chicken Salad Lettuce Wraps with Homemade Mayonnaise, 103

D

Dairy products, 10

Dates
- Apple Walnut Bars, 115
- Banana Chocolate Tart, 204–205
- Rich Chocolate Fudge, 207

Desserts, 195–209
- Apple Crisp with Fresh Ginger, 200–201
- Banana Chocolate Tart, 204–205
- Banana Maple Nut "Ice Cream," 197
- Berry Crumb Cake, 202–203
- Cocoa Almond Pudding, 198
- Mini Cheesecakes in Caramel Sauce, 208–209

Molten Chocolate Cakes, 206
Peanut Butter Oatmeal Cookies, 199
Rich Chocolate Fudge, 207
Yogurt Blueberry Ice Pops, 196
Dining out, tips for, 227–228
Dirty dozen, 21
Doubling of recipe, 142

E

Edens Foods, 19
Eggplant, Stacked, Parmesan, 128–129
Eggs
Bacon-Crusted Mini Quiches with Mushrooms and Greens, 84–85
Breakfast Tacos with Green Chiles, Goat Cheese, and Salsa Verde, 79–80
Brussels Sprouts Hash with Caramelized Onions and Poached Eggs, 148–149
Egg Salad Sandwich with Greek Yogurt and Dill, 102
Fresh Herb Frittata with Peas, Bacon, and Feta Cheese, 88–89
Mini Cheesecakes in Caramel Sauce, 208–209
Poached Eggs and Asparagus on Whole-Grain Toast, 82–83
Poached Eggs in Spicy Tomato Sauce, 81
Pork Fried Brown Rice with Pineapple and Cashews, 186–187
Red Pepper, Spinach, and Goat Cheese Frittata Bites, 76
Scrambled Egg, Goat Cheese, and Cherry Tomato Pita Sandwich, 77–78
Egg whites
Scrambled Egg, Goat Cheese, and Cherry Tomato Pita Sandwich, 77–78

Enchiladas
Chicken Enchiladas Verdes with Goat Cheese, 168–169
Spinach and White Bean Enchiladas with Cashew Cheese, 135–136
Endosperm, 3
Energy, boosting your, 2
Environmental Working Group, 21

F

Fats, healthful, 10
Feta cheese
Balsamic-Roasted Vegetables with Quinoa, 139–140
Fresh Herb Frittata with Peas, Bacon, and Feta Cheese, 88–89
Goat Cheese and Spinach-Stuffed Pork Chops, 181–182
Mediterranean Chickpea Salad with Red Bell Peppers and Feta Cheese, 94
Whole-Wheat Pasta with Chickpeas and Spicy Tomato Sauce, 143
Fiber, 2
Fish and Seafood, 151–163
Balsamic-Glazed Wild Salmon with Garlicky Sautéed Spinach, 157–158
Garlic-Broiled Shrimp and Peppers over Quinoa, 154–155
Grilled Shrimp Tacos with Salsa Verde and Spicy Slaw, 152–153
Italian Fish Stew, 163
Oven-Roasted Monkfish and Asparagus with Romesco Sauce, 160
Red Snapper with Spiced Pumpkin Seed Butter, 159
Seared Ahi Tuna with Chili-Lime Aioli, 156

Soy-Glaze Cod with Japanese-Style Pickled Cucumber, 161–162
Flash-freezing, 19
Food labels, learning to read, 18, 20
Foods to avoid, 10–12
Free radicals, 3
Fresh Basil Pesto, 219
Pesto White Bean Spread, 124
Roasted Vegetable Pitas with Pesto Mayonnaise, 101
Turkey Meatballs with Whole-Wheat Spaghetti and Spicy Tomato Sauce, 177–178
Fresh Herb Frittata with Peas, Bacon, and Feta Cheese, 88–89
Freshness, 19
Fried rice, 186
Pork Fried Brown Rice with Pineapple and Cashews, 186–187
Frittata
Fresh Herb Frittata with Peas, Bacon, and Feta Cheese, 88–89
Red Pepper, Spinach, and Goat Cheese Frittata Bites, 76
Fruits, fresh, 1–2, 8, 13–14. *See also specific*

G

Garden Salad with Chicken and Balsamic Vinaigrette, 100
Garlic-Broiled Shrimp and Peppers over Quinoa, 154–155
Ginger Berry Smoothie, 60
Goat cheese
Breakfast Tacos with Green Chiles, Goat Cheese, and Salsa Verde, 79–80
Chicken Enchiladas Verdes with Goat Cheese, 168–169
Goat Cheese and Spinach-Stuffed Pork Chops, 181–182
Red Pepper, Spinach, and Goat Cheese Frittata Bites, 76

Roasted Butternut Squash and
  Black Bean Burritos with
  Goat Cheese, 137–138
Roasted Butternut Squash
  Salad with Goat Cheese,
  Walnuts, and Balsamic
  Vinaigrette, 92–93
Roasted Vegetable Pitas with
  Pesto Mayonnaise, 101
Scrambled Egg, Goat Cheese,
  and Cherry Tomato Pita
  Sandwich, 77–78
Granola
  Homemade Cinnamon
    Granola, 61–62
Greek yogurt. *See also* Yogurt
  Apple Crisp with Fresh Ginger,
    200–201
  Egg Salad Sandwich with
    Greek Yogurt and Dill, 102
  Lamb Loin Chops with Yogurt-
    Mint Sauce, 179–180
  Mini Cheesecakes in Caramel
    Sauce, 208–209
  Yogurt Blueberry Ice Pops, 196
Green beans
  Spicy Black Bean Soup with
    Vegetables, 108–109
Grilled Pineapple and Pork
  Skewers, 183
Grilled Shrimp Tacos with Salsa
  Verde and Spicy Slaw, 152–153
Grilling, 26
Ground beef
  Bacon-Wrapped Meatloaf,
    188–189
Guacamole, 212

H

Halibut
  Italian Fish Stew, 163
Herbs, 9. *See also specific*
Heterocyclic amines (HCAs), 26
Homemade Almond Milk, 225
Homemade Cinnamon Granola,
  61–62
Homemade Mayonnaise, 217

Curried Chicken Salad Lettuce
  Wraps with Homemade
  Mayonnaise, 103
Egg Salad Sandwich with
  Greek Yogurt and Dill, 102
Roasted Vegetable Pitas with
  Pesto Mayonnaise, 101
Seared Ahi Tuna with Chili-
  Lime Aioli, 156
Thai-Style Curried Chicken
  Burgers, 174
Honey Sesame Crackers, 118
Hydrogenated fats, 11

I

Immunity, strengthening your, 2
Ingredients, list of, 20
In-season foods, 8
Iron, 2
Italian Fish Stew, 163

J

Jalapeño peppers
  Grilled Shrimp Tacos with
    Salsa Verde and Spicy Slaw,
    152–153
  Pico de Gallo, 213
  Roasted Butternut Squash and
    Black Bean Burritos with
    Goat Cheese, 137–138
  Salsa Verde, 218
  Seared Ahi Tuna with Chili-
    Lime Aioli, 156
  Spiced Chicken Wraps with
    Yogurt Dressing and Fresh
    Mint, 104
  Spicy Black Bean Soup with
    Vegetables, 108–109
  Spicy Southwestern Corn and
    Bean Salad, 91
  Vegetarian Chili with Pinto
    Beans, 130–131

K

Kitchen Staples, 211–226
  Balsamic Vinaigrette, 214
  Cashew Cheese, 224

Chicken Broth, 222
Fresh Basil Pesto, 219
Guacamole, 212
Homemade Almond Milk, 225
Homemade Mayonnaise, 217
Lemon Vinaigrette, 215
Pico de Gallo, 213
Romesco Sauce, 220
Salsa Verde, 218
Spicy Tomato Sauce, 221
Vegetable Broth, 223
Whipped Coconut
  Cream, 226
Yogurt Dressing, 216
Korean Pork Lettuce Wraps with
  Fresh Herbs, 105
Korean Stir-Fried Pork with
  Brown Rice, 184–185

L

Lamb Loin Chops with Yogurt-
  Mint Sauce, 179–180
Legumes, 9
Lemon Vinaigrette, 215
  Brown Rice and Black Bean
    Salad with Spinach and
    Lemon Vinaigrette, 97
  Brussels Sprouts and
    Chickpea Salad with Dried
    Cranberries, 95
  Quinoa Salad with Cannellini
    Beans, Tomatoes, and
    Lemon Vinaigrette, 96
Lentils
  Smoky Red Lentil Soup with
    Greens, 106–107
Lettuce
  Chickpea Tostadas with
    Cashew Cheese, 133–134
  Curried Chicken Salad Lettuce
    Wraps with Homemade
    Mayonnaise, 103
  Garden Salad with Chicken
    and Balsamic
    Vinaigrette, 100
  Korean Pork Lettuce Wraps
    with Fresh Herbs, 105

Roasted Butternut Squash Salad with Goat Cheese, Walnuts, and Balsamic Vinaigrette, 92–93
Roasted Vegetable Pitas with Pesto Mayonnaise, 101
Shrimp Salad over Greens with Yogurt Dressing, 98
Thai-Style Curried Chicken Burgers, 174
Limes
  Grilled Shrimp Tacos with Salsa Verde and Spicy Slaw, 152–153
  Pico de Gallo, 213
  Salsa Verde, 218
Lunch, 87–109
  Brown Rice and Black Bean Salad with Spinach and Lemon Vinaigrette, 97
  Brussels Sprouts and Chickpea Salad with Dried Cranberries, 95
  Caprese Salad with Balsamic Vinaigrette, 90
  Curried Chicken Salad Lettuce Wraps with Homemade Mayonnaise, 103
  Egg Salad Sandwich with Greek Yogurt and Dill, 102
  Fresh Herb Frittata with Peas, Bacon, and Feta Cheese, 88–89
  Garden Salad with Chicken and Balsamic Vinaigrette, 100
  Korean Pork Lettuce Wraps with Fresh Herbs, 105
  Mediterranean Chickpea Salad with Red Bell Peppers and Feta Cheese, 94
  Quinoa Salad with Cannellini Beans, Tomatoes, and Lemon Vinaigrette, 96
  Roasted Butternut Squash Salad with Goat Cheese, Walnuts, and Balsamic Vinaigrette, 92–93
  Roasted Vegetable Pitas with Pesto Mayonnaise, 101
  Shrimp Salad over Greens with Yogurt Dressing, 98
  Smoky Red Lentil Soup with Greens, 106–107
  Spiced Chicken Wraps with Yogurt Dressing and Fresh Mint, 104
  Spicy Black Bean Soup with Vegetables, 108–109
  Spicy Southwestern Corn and Bean Salad, 91
  Spinach Salad with Chicken and Sun-Dried Tomatoes and Basil Vinaigrette, 99

M

Meal plans, 17–29
  getting most out of, 17–18
  week four, 51–56
  week one, 33–38
  week three, 45–50
  week two, 39–44
Meals, eating small, 6
Meat and Poultry Dinners, 165–193
  Bacon-Wrapped Meatloaf, 188–189
  Chicken and White Bean Chili, 175–176
  Chicken Enchiladas Verdes with Goat Cheese, 168–169
  Goat Cheese and Spinach-Stuffed Pork Chops, 181–182
  Grilled Pineapple and Pork Skewers, 183
  Korean Stir-Fried Pork with Brown Rice, 184–185
  Lamb Loin Chops with Yogurt-Mint Sauce, 179–180
  Pork Fried Brown Rice with Pineapple and Cashews, 186–187
  Quinoa Fried "Rice" with Flank Steak and Peas, 192–193
  Roasted Chicken and Vegetables, 166–167
  Roasted Chicken Breasts with Mustard and Greens, 172–173
  Sesame-Soy Marinated Flank Steak with Wasabi-Spiked Cauliflower Purée, 190–191
  Tandoori-Spiced Chicken Breast with Crisp Cucumber Salad, 170–171
  Thai-Style Curried Chicken Burgers, 174
  Turkey Meatballs with Whole-Wheat Spaghetti and Spicy Tomato Sauce, 177–178
Meatballs, Turkey, with Whole-Wheat Spaghetti and Spicy Tomato Sauce, 177–178
Meatloaf, Bacon-Wrapped, 188–189
Mediterranean Chickpea Salad with Red Bell Peppers and Feta Cheese, 94
Medium-chain triglycerides (MCTs), 23
Microwaving, 27
Milk substitutes, 10
Mini Cheesecakes in Caramel Sauce, 208–209
Mint
  Korean Pork Lettuce Wraps with Fresh Herbs, 105
  Lamb Loin Chops with Yogurt-Mint Sauce, 179–180
  Spiced Chicken Wraps with Yogurt Dressing and Fresh Mint, 104
Molten Chocolate Cakes, 206

Monkfish, Oven-Roasted, and Asparagus with Romesco Sauce, 160
Mozzarella cheese
  Caprese Salad with Balsamic Vinaigrette, 90
  Stacked Eggplant Parmesan, 128–129
Muffins, Whole-Wheat Blueberry, with Cinnamon-Sugar Topping, 70–71
Muir Glen, 19
Mushrooms
  Bacon-Crusted Mini Quiches with Mushrooms and Greens, 84–85
  Balsamic-Roasted Vegetables with Quinoa, 139–140
  Risotto with Mushrooms and Peas, 146–147

N

No-Bake Coconut Granola Bars, 63–64
Nondairy milks, 10
Nutrition facts, 20
Nuts, 9. *See also specific*

O

Oat flour
  Banana Blueberry Whole-Grain Pancakes, 74–75
Oats, 2
  Apple Crisp with Fresh Ginger, 200–201
  Apple Walnut Bars, 115
  Homemade Cinnamon Granola, 61–62
  No-Bake Coconut Granola Bars, 63–64
  Overnight Cinnamon Oatmeal, 65
  Peanut Butter Energy Bites, 113
  Peanut Butter Oatmeal Cookies, 199
  Sweet Quinoa Breakfast Cups, 72–73
Organic foods, 1, 21

Oven-Baked Sweet Potato Fries, 123
Oven-Roasted Monkfish and Asparagus with Romesco Sauce, 160
Overnight Cinnamon Oatmeal, 65

P

Packaged foods
  avoiding, 10
  choosing whole foods over, 5
Paleo diet, comparing with clean eating, 4
Pancakes
  Banana Blueberry Whole-Grain Pancakes, 74–75
  Protein-Packed Freezer Waffles (or Pancakes), 66–67
Pantry, stocking your, 22, 36–37, 42–43, 48–49, 54–55
Peanut butter
  Creamy Peanut Butter–Yogurt Dip, 119
  Peanut Butter Energy Bites, 113
  Peanut Butter Oatmeal Cookies, 199
  Rich Chocolate Fudge, 207
Peas
  Fresh Herb Frittata with Peas, Bacon, and Feta Cheese, 88–89
  Quinoa Fried "Rice" with Flank Steak and Peas, 192–193
  Risotto with Mushrooms and Peas, 146–147
Peppers. *See* Jalapeño peppers; Red bell peppers; Yellow bell peppers
Pesto White Bean Spread, 124
Pico de Gallo, 213
Pineapple
  Grilled Pineapple and Pork Skewers, 183
  Pineapple Coconut Trail Mix, 112

Pork Fried Brown Rice with Pineapple and Cashews, 186–187
  Tropical Sweet Bars, 114
Pinto Beans, Vegetarian Chili with, 130–131
Pitas
  Roasted Vegetable Pitas with Pesto Mayonnaise, 101
  Scrambled Egg, Goat Cheese, and Cherry Tomato Pita Sandwich, 77–78
Plum tomatoes
  Pico de Gallo, 213
Poached Eggs and Asparagus on Whole-Grain Toast, 82–83
Poached Eggs in Spicy Tomato Sauce, 81
Poaching, 26
Polycylic aromatic hydrocarbons (PAHs), 26–27
Pork
  Bacon-Wrapped Meatloaf, 188–189
  Goat Cheese and Spinach-Stuffed Pork Chops, 181–182
  Grilled Pineapple and Pork Skewers, 183
  Korean Pork Lettuce Wraps with Fresh Herbs, 105
  Korean Stir-Fried Pork with Brown Rice, 184–185
  Pork Fried Brown Rice with Pineapple and Cashews, 186–187
Portions, 6–7
Potatoes. *See also* Sweet potatoes
  Roasted Chicken and Vegetables, 166–167
Processed foods, eliminating from diet, 1
Protein-Packed Freezer Waffles (or Pancakes), 66–67
Proteins, lean, 10
Pumpkin, 19
  Pumpkin and Chickpea Curry, 132

Pumpkin seeds
    Red Snapper with Spiced Pumpkin Seed Butter, 159

Q

Quiches, Bacon-Crusted Mini, with Mushrooms and Greens, 84–85
Quinoa
    Balsamic-Roasted Vegetables with Quinoa, 139–140
    Garlic-Broiled Shrimp and Peppers over Quinoa, 154–155
    Quinoa Fried "Rice" with Flank Steak and Peas, 192–193
    Quinoa Salad with Cannellini Beans, Tomatoes, and Lemon Vinaigrette, 96
    Quinoa-Stuffed Peppers with Black Beans and Yogurt Dressing, 141–142
    Sweet Quinoa Breakfast Cups, 72–73

R

Raisins
    Rich Chocolate Fudge, 207
Red bell peppers
    Bacon-Wrapped Meatloaf, 188–189
    Garlic-Broiled Shrimp and Peppers over Quinoa, 154–155
    Korean Stir-Fried Pork with Brown Rice, 184–185
    Mediterranean Chickpea Salad with Red Bell Peppers and Feta Cheese, 94
    Quinoa-Stuffed Peppers with Black Beans and Yogurt Dressing, 141–142
    Red Pepper, Spinach, and Goat Cheese Frittata Bites, 76
    Romesco Sauce, 220
    Thai-Style Curried Chicken Burgers, 174
    Vegetable Stew, 144–145
    Vegetarian Chili with Pinto Beans, 130–131
Red Snapper with Spiced Pumpkin Seed Butter, 159
Refined flour, 13
Refined grains, 11, 20
Refined sugar, avoiding, 4, 5, 11, 20
Rice. See Arborio rice; Brown rice
Rich Chocolate Fudge, 207
Risotto with Mushrooms and Peas, 146–147
Roasted Butternut Squash and Black Bean Burritos with Goat Cheese, 137–138
Roasted Butternut Squash Salad with Goat Cheese, Walnuts, and Balsamic Vinaigrette, 92–93
Roasted Chicken and Vegetables, 166–167
Roasted Chicken Breasts with Mustard and Greens, 172–173
Roasted Vegetable Pitas with Pesto Mayonnaise, 101
Roasting, 25
Romesco Sauce, 220
    Oven-Roasted Monkfish and Asparagus with Romesco Sauce, 160

S

Salads
    Brussels Sprouts and Chickpea Salad with Dried Cranberries, 95
    Caprese Salad with Balsamic Vinaigrette, 90
    Curried Chicken Salad Lettuce Wraps with Homemade Mayonnaise, 103
    Garden Salad with Chicken and Balsamic Vinaigrette, 100
    Mediterranean Chickpea Salad with Red Bell Peppers and Feta Cheese, 94
    Quinoa Salad with Cannellini Beans, Tomatoes, and Lemon Vinaigrette, 96
    Roasted Butternut Squash Salad with Goat Cheese, Walnuts, and Balsamic Vinaigrette, 92–93
    Shrimp Salad over Greens with Yogurt Dressing, 98
    Spicy Southwestern Corn and Bean Salad, 91
    Spinach Salad with Chicken and Sun-Dried Tomatoes and Basil Vinaigrette, 99
    Tandoori-Spiced Chicken Breast with Crisp Cucumber Salad, 170–171
Salmon, Balsamic-Glazed Wild, with Garlicky Sautéed Spinach, 157–158
Salsa
    Chickpea Tostadas with Cashew Cheese, 133–134
    Pico de Gallo, 213
Salsa Verde, 218
    Breakfast Tacos with Green Chiles, Goat Cheese, and Salsa Verde, 79–80
    Chicken Enchiladas Verdes with Goat Cheese, 168–169
    Grilled Shrimp Tacos with Salsa Verde and Spicy Slaw, 152–153
Salt, avoiding excess, 5
Sandwiches. See also Wraps
    Egg Salad Sandwich with Greek Yogurt and Dill, 102
    Scrambled Egg, Goat Cheese, and Cherry Tomato Pita Sandwich, 77–78
Saturated fats, avoiding, 3, 5, 11, 20
Sautéing, 26

Index 243

Scrambled Egg, Goat Cheese, and Cherry Tomato Pita Sandwich, 77–78
Seared Ahi Tuna with Chili-Lime Aioli, 156
Seeds, 9. *See also* Pumpkin seeds; Sesame seeds
Serving, appearance of, 7
Sesame seeds
    Honey Sesame Crackers, 118
    Sesame-Soy Marinated Flank Steak with Wasabi-Spiked Cauliflower Purée, 190–191
Shopping list, 37–38, 43, 49, 55
Shopping tips, 22
Shrimp
    Garlic-Broiled Shrimp and Peppers over Quinoa, 154–155
    Grilled Shrimp Tacos with Salsa Verde and Spicy Slaw, 152–153
    Shrimp Salad over Greens with Yogurt Dressing, 98
Smoky Red Lentil Soup with Greens, 106–107
Smoky-Sweet Chili Almonds, 121
Smoothies, Ginger Berry, 60
Snacks, 111–124
    Apple Walnut Bars, 115
    Banana Nut Bread, 116–117
    Basil Garlic Zucchini Chips, 122
    Creamy Peanut Butter–Yogurt Dip, 119
    Honey Sesame Crackers, 118
    Oven-Baked Sweet Potato Fries, 123
    Peanut Butter Energy Bites, 113
    Pesto White Bean Spread, 124
    Pineapple Coconut Trail Mix, 112
    Smoky-Sweet Chili Almonds, 121
    Spiced Roasted Chickpeas, 120
    Tropical Sweet Bars, 114
Soluble fiber, 3

Soups. *See also* Stews
    Smoky Red Lentil Soup with Greens, 106–107
    Spicy Black Bean Soup with Vegetables, 108–109
    Soy-Glaze Cod with Japanese-Style Pickled Cucumber, 161–162
Spiced Chicken Wraps with Yogurt Dressing and Fresh Mint, 104
Spiced Roasted Chickpeas, 120
Spices, 9. *See also specific*
Spicy Black Bean Soup with Vegetables, 108–109
Spicy Southwestern Corn and Bean Salad, 91
Spicy Tomato Sauce, 221
    Poached Eggs in Spicy Tomato Sauce, 81
    Stacked Eggplant Parmesan, 128–129
    Turkey Meatballs with Whole-Wheat Spaghetti and Spicy Tomato Sauce, 177–178
    Whole-Wheat Pasta with Chickpeas and Spicy Tomato Sauce, 143
Spinach
    Balsamic-Glazed Wild Salmon with Garlicky Sautéed Spinach, 157–158
    Brown Rice and Black Bean Salad with Spinach and Lemon Vinaigrette, 97
    Egg Salad Sandwich with Greek Yogurt and Dill, 102
    Goat Cheese and Spinach-Stuffed Pork Chops, 181–182
    Quinoa-Stuffed Peppers with Black Beans and Yogurt Dressing, 141–142
    Red Pepper, Spinach, and Goat Cheese Frittata Bites, 76
    Smoky Red Lentil Soup with Greens, 106–107

Spinach and White Bean Enchiladas with Cashew Cheese, 135–136
Spinach Salad with Chicken and Sun-Dried Tomatoes and Basil Vinaigrette, 99
Stacked Eggplant Parmesan, 128–129
Steaming, 26
Stew, Italian Fish, 163
Stir-frying, 26
    Korean Stir-Fried Pork with Brown Rice, 184–185
Strawberries
    Ginger Berry Smoothie, 60
Sun-dried tomatoes
    Goat Cheese and Spinach-Stuffed Pork Chops, 181–182
    Spinach Salad with Chicken and Sun-Dried Tomatoes and Basil Vinaigrette, 99
Sweeteners, 20
Sweet potatoes
    Oven-Baked Sweet Potato Fries, 123
    Spicy Black Bean Soup with Vegetables, 108–109
Sweet Quinoa Breakfast Cups, 72–73
Swiss chard
    Bacon-Crusted Mini Quiches with Mushrooms and Greens, 84–85
    Roasted Chicken Breasts with Mustard and Greens, 172–173

T

Tacos
    Breakfast Tacos with Green Chiles, Goat Cheese, and Salsa Verde, 79–80
    Grilled Shrimp Tacos with Salsa Verde and Spicy Slaw, 152–153
    Tandoori-Spiced Chicken Breast with Crisp Cucumber Salad, 170–171

Thai-Style Curried Chicken Burgers, 174
Tip to double the recipe, 80
Tofu
   Banana Chocolate Tart, 204–205
   Ginger Berry Smoothie, 60
   Protein-Packed Freezer Waffles (or Pancakes), 66–67
Tomatillos
   Salsa Verde, 218
Tomatoes, 19. *See also* Cherry tomatoes; Plum tomatoes; Sun-dried tomatoes
   Caprese Salad with Balsamic Vinaigrette, 90
   Egg Salad Sandwich with Greek Yogurt and Dill, 102
   Garden Salad with Chicken and Balsamic Vinaigrette, 100
   Guacamole, 212
   Italian Fish Stew, 163
   Pumpkin and Chickpea Curry, 132
   Quinoa Salad with Cannellini Beans, Tomatoes, and Lemon Vinaigrette, 96
   Quinoa-Stuffed Peppers with Black Beans and Yogurt Dressing, 141–142
   Smoky Red Lentil Soup with Greens, 106–107
   Spicy Southwestern Corn and Bean Salad, 91
   Spicy Tomato Sauce, 221
   Thai-Style Curried Chicken Burgers, 174
   Vegetable Stew, 144–145
   Vegetarian Chili with Pinto Beans, 130–131
Tools and equipment, 25
Tortillas
   Breakfast Tacos with Green Chiles, Goat Cheese, and Salsa Verde, 79–80
   Chicken Enchiladas Verdes with Goat Cheese, 168–169
   Chickpea Tostadas with Cashew Cheese, 133–134
   Grilled Shrimp Tacos with Salsa Verde and Spicy Slaw, 152–153
   Roasted Butternut Squash and Black Bean Burritos with Goat Cheese, 137–138
   Spiced Chicken Wraps with Yogurt Dressing and Fresh Mint, 104
   Spinach and White Bean Enchiladas with Cashew Cheese, 135–136
Trader Joe's, 19
Trans fats, avoiding, 3, 5, 11, 20
Tropical Sweet Bars, 114
Tuna
   Seared Ahi Tuna with Chili-Lime Aioli, 156
Turkey Meatballs with Whole-Wheat Spaghetti and Spicy Tomato Sauce, 177–178

V

Vegetable Broth, 223
   Garlic-Broiled Shrimp and Peppers over Quinoa, 154–155
   Risotto with Mushrooms and Peas, 146–147
   Smoky Red Lentil Soup with Greens, 106–107
   Spicy Black Bean Soup with Vegetables, 108–109
Vegetable Stew, 144–145
Vegetables, fresh, 1–2, 9, 13–14. *See also specific*
Vegetarian Chili with Pinto Beans, 130–131
Vegetarian diet, 13
Vegetarian Dinners, 127–149
   Balsamic-Roasted Vegetables with Quinoa, 139–140
   Brussels Sprouts Hash with Caramelized Onions and Poached Eggs, 148–149
   Chickpea Tostadas with Cashew Cheese, 133–134
   Pumpkin and Chickpea Curry, 132
   Quinoa-Stuffed Peppers with Black Beans and Yogurt Dressing, 141–142
   Risotto with Mushrooms and Peas, 146–147
   Roasted Butternut Squash and Black Bean Burritos with Goat Cheese, 137–138
   Spinach and White Bean Enchiladas with Cashew Cheese, 135–136
   Stacked Eggplant Parmesan, 128–129
   Vegetable Stew, 144–145
   Vegetarian Chili with Pinto Beans, 130–131
   Whole-Wheat Pasta with Chickpeas and Spicy Tomato Sauce, 143
Vinaigrette. *See also* Lemon Vinaigrette
   Caprese Salad with Balsamic Vinaigrette, 90
   Roasted Butternut Squash Salad with Goat Cheese, Walnuts, and Balsamic Vinaigrette, 92–93

W

Waffles, Protein-Packed Freezer (or Pancakes), 66–67
Walnuts
   Apple Walnut Bars, 115
   Banana Maple Nut "Ice Cream," 197
   Banana Nut Bread, 116–117
   Fresh Basil Pesto, 219
   No-Bake Coconut Granola Bars, 63–64
Water, drinking plenty of, 6

Weight loss, 2
Wheat flour, 20
Whipped Coconut Cream, 226
White fish
   Italian Fish Stew, 163
Whole Foods, 19
Whole foods, choosing over packaged foods, 5
Whole-grain bread
   Egg Salad Sandwich with Greek Yogurt and Dill, 102
   Poached Eggs and Asparagus on Whole-Grain Toast, 82–83
   Poached Eggs in Spicy Tomato Sauce, 81
Whole-grain flours, 13
Whole grains, 1, 2, 3, 9
Whole-wheat flour
   Banana Blueberry Whole-Grain Pancakes, 74–75
   Banana Nut Bread, 116–117
   Protein-Packed Freezer Waffles (or Pancakes), 66–67
   Whole-Wheat Blueberry Muffins with Cinnamon-Sugar Topping, 70–71
   Whole-Wheat Maple Cinnamon Rolls, 68–69
Whole-wheat pasta
   Turkey Meatballs with Whole-Wheat Spaghetti and Spicy Tomato Sauce, 177–178
   Whole-Wheat Pasta with Chickpeas and Spicy Tomato Sauce, 143
Wraps. *See also* Sandwiches
   Curried Chicken Salad Lettuce Wraps with Homemade Mayonnaise, 103
   Korean Pork Lettuce Wraps with Fresh Herbs, 105
   Spiced Chicken Wraps with Yogurt Dressing and Fresh Mint, 104

Y

Yeast
   Cashew Cheese, 224
   Fresh Basil Pesto, 219
   Whole-Wheat Maple Cinnamon Rolls, 68–69
Yellow bell peppers
   Balsamic-Roasted Vegetables with Quinoa, 139–140
   Korean Stir-Fried Pork with Brown Rice, 184–185
   Thai-Style Curried Chicken Burgers, 174
Yogurt. *See also* Greek yogurt
   Apple Crisp with Fresh Ginger, 200–201
   Creamy Peanut Butter–Yogurt Dip, 119
   Tandoori-Spiced Chicken Breast with Crisp Cucumber Salad, 170–171
   Yogurt Blueberry Ice Pops, 196
   Yogurt Dressing, 216
Yogurt Dressing, 216
   Quinoa-Stuffed Peppers with Black Beans and Yogurt Dressing, 141–142
   Shrimp Salad over Greens with Yogurt Dressing, 98
   Spiced Chicken Wraps with Yogurt Dressing and Fresh Mint, 104

Z

Zucchini
   Balsamic-Roasted Vegetables with Quinoa, 139–140
   Basil Garlic Zucchini Chips, 122